Colleen McLaughlin
Sharlene Swartz
Susan Kiragu
Shelina Walli
Mussa Mohamed

GW00506591

Old enough to know

Consulting children about sex and AIDS education in Africa

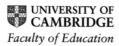

UNIVERSITY OF CAMBRIDGE
Faculty of Education

HSRC PRESS

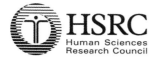 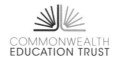 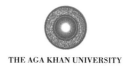

HSRC
Human Sciences
Research Council

THE CENTRE FOR
COMMONWEALTH EDUCATION

COMMONWEALTH
EDUCATION TRUST

THE AGA KHAN UNIVERSITY

Published by HSRC Press
Private Bag X9182, Cape Town, 8000, South Africa
www.hsrcpress.ac.za

First published 2012

ISBN (soft cover): 978-0-7969-2374-5
ISBN (pdf): 978-0-7969-2375-2
ISBN (e-pub): 978-0-7969-2376-9

Copyedited by Mark Ronan
Typeset by Nazley Samsodien
Cover design by Michelle Staples

Printed and bound by Unity Press, 57 Mobile Road, Airport Industria, Cape Town

Distributed in Africa by Blue Weaver
Tel: +27 (0) 21 701 4477; Fax: +27 (0) 21 701 7302
www.oneworldbooks.com

Distributed in Europe and the United Kingdom by Eurospan Distribution Services (EDS)
Tel: +44 (0) 17 6760 4972; Fax: +44 (0) 17 6760 1640
www.eurospanbookstore.com

Distributed in North America by River North Editions, from IPG
Call toll-free: (800) 888 4741; Fax: +1 (312) 337 5985
www.ipgbook.com

Contents

Tables and figures

TABLES

FIGURES

Acknowledgments

We would like to thank the individuals and organisations that enabled this research to take place. The researchers came from three organisations and we thank them: The Centre for Commonwealth Education, Faculty of Education, University of Cambridge, UK, which funded the research; the Human Sciences Research Council, Cape Town, South Africa, and the Aga Khan University Institute for Educational Development (East Africa), Dar es Salaam, Tanzania. We would also like to thank Duncan Scott and Busi Magazi at the Human Sciences Research Council, who gave of their time and effort in collecting and managing the data and contributing to the writing, as did Mary Cobbett at the Commonwealth Centre, who helped in the final stages. We thank the ministries and departments of education in Kenya, South Africa and Tanzania for giving permission for this research. We owe the greatest thanks to the students and teachers in the schools we worked in. Research makes great demands on colleagues in schools and we are grateful for their time and cooperation.

Abbreviations and acronyms

ABC	Abstain, Be faithful, Condomise
AIDS	Acquired immune deficiency syndrome
AMREF	Africa Medical and Research Foundation
ARV	Antiretroviral
ASKAIDS	African Sexual Knowledges (research project)
CRE	Christian religion education
FGD	Focus group discussion
HIV	Human immunodeficiency virus
HSRC	Human Sciences Research Council
IRF	Initiation, response, follow-up
KANCO	Kenya AIDS NGOs Consortium
NGO	Non-governmental organisation
UN	United Nations
UNAIDS	Joint United Nations Programme on HIV/AIDS
UNESCO	United Nations Education, Scientific and Cultural Organization
UNICEF	United Nations Children's (Emergency) Fund

Foreword

The Centre for Commonwealth Education (CCE) at the University of Cambridge's Faculty of Education began in 2007. Its aim was to make a vibrant and long term contribution to primary and secondary education, and to initial and continuing teacher education, throughout the Commonwealth. Over the past five years it has done so through a number of strategic projects throughout the world. Its guiding principle has been to build sustainable partnerships which aim to understand and increase young people's and teachers' participation in their own learning and to explore how that learning extends beyond schooling, how it connects with prior learning, and with other arenas of learning in informal as well as formal contexts. The ultimate goal is to improve the quality of children's lives, to enrich the quality of learning and teaching, and to improve the well-being of children and youth within and beyond school.

The work of the CCE is premised on listening to students, teachers, school leaders, local and national policy makers and related agencies so as to develop intervention strategies which are sensitive to local needs and to broader cultural issues while, at the same time able to offer constructive challenge in a spirit of collaborative inquiry. Research is thus integral, ongoing and formative, serving to build capacity not only of the Centre but of schools and agencies engaged with us in this work.

I am exceptionally pleased that our study conducted in Tanzania, Kenya and South Africa with local partners has resulted in this important publication. *Old enough to know* is an innovative exploration of what children think about sex and AIDS and what they want to know and learn. It provides the outcome of the researchers' consultation with pupils around their knowledge of sexuality, and shows in technicolour, children's (almost) daily confrontation and/or experimentation with sexuality in their living environments. This book offers an important contribution towards understanding how children's sexual subjectivity is shaped by contexts of culture, gender, poverty, home environments and schooling. The study offers possibilities to resolve the gap between children's everyday realities on the one hand and teachers' curriculum-based and cultural restraints on the other.

Old enough to know is a profound study, and significantly advances both our knowledge base and our methodological arsenal. It provides a clearly structured and coherent story for the reader that delves into difficult areas. It includes theoretical constructs that are introduced when necessary, to structure and develop pertinent arguments, and the use of children's own words gives added power and attraction to the narrative, and increases readability. The authors also showcase innovative, child-friendly, participative research methods. The ways of working, the detail with which this is set out, and the appendices detailing specific activities employed in the study, will prove invaluable to other researchers in the field, and will make a significant contribution to the development of qualitative research amongst vulnerable children.

I wholeheartedly recommend this book to those interested in innovative research methodologies which have applicability in terms of accessing student voice and those interested in research methodologies appropriate to research contexts in the South (with particular applicability to controversial issues). Equally, those interested in the HIV and AIDS education debate will find the text ground-breaking and wide-ranging and with the potential to make a very significant and compelling contribution to implementing an educational social vaccine against the epidemic.

Mike Younger

Mike Younger
Director of the Centre for Commonwealth Education
University of Cambridge Faculty of Education

Old enough to know visual data: Photovoice

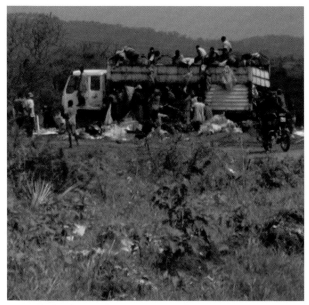

1   Rubbish dump near School A, Kenya

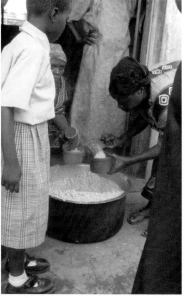

2   Feeding programme, School C, Kenya

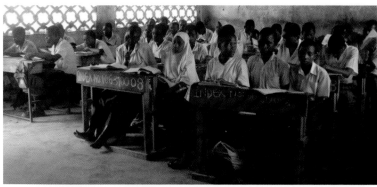

3   Primary school classroom in Kenya

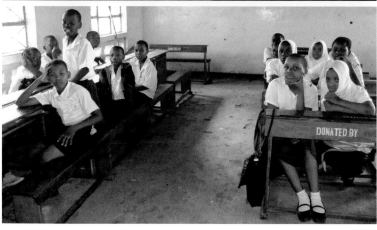

4   Primary school classroom in Tanzania

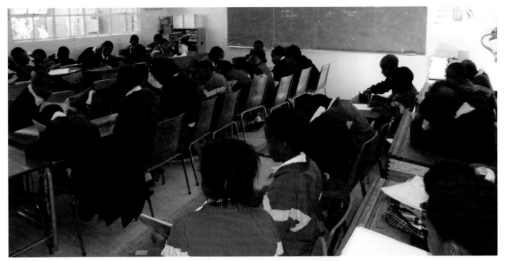

5 Primary school classroom in South Africa

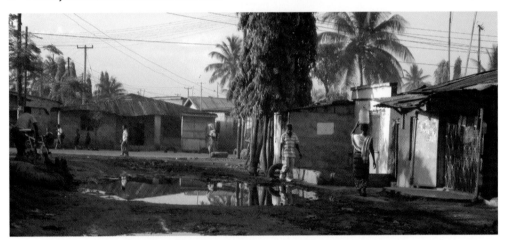

6 Children's neighbourhood, Tanzania

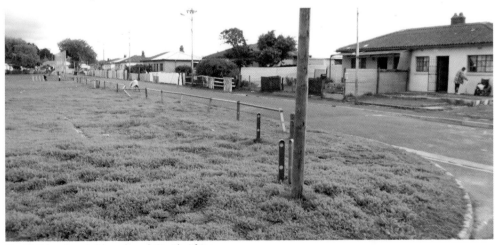

7 Children's neighbourhood, South Africa

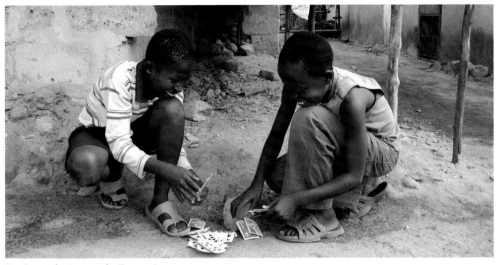

8 Boys playing cards, Tanzania

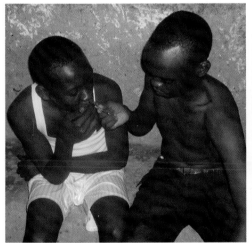

9 Boys smoking marijuana, Kenya

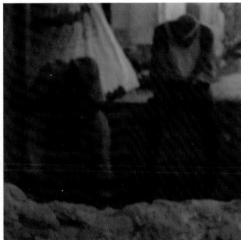

10 Effect of taking drugs, Kenya

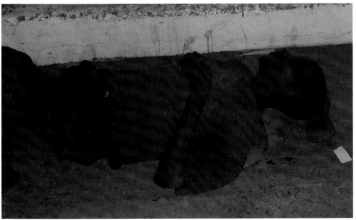

11 Male youth passed out after taking drugs, Kenya

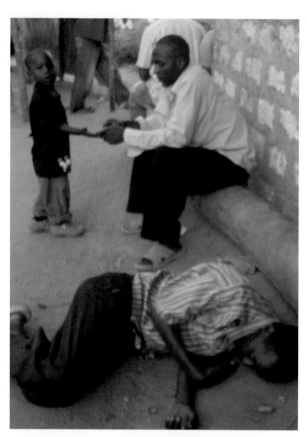

12 Outside a beer den/brothel, Kenya

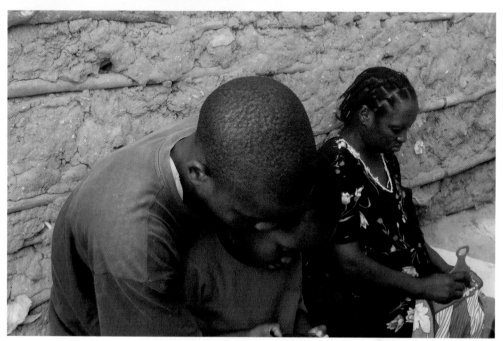

13 Alleged public fondling in the presence of children, Kenya

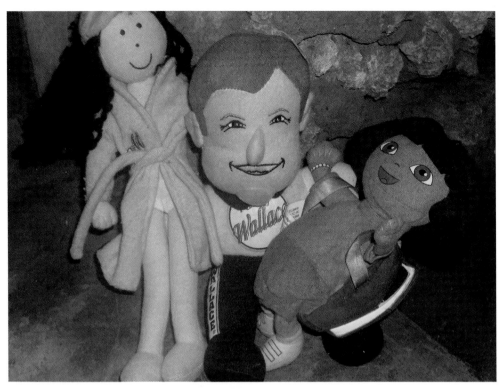

14 Portrayal of sex for money by two girls, Kenya

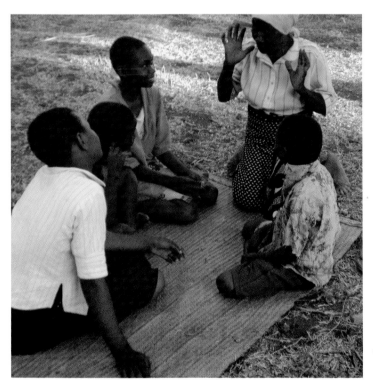

15 Grandmother talking to children, Tanzania

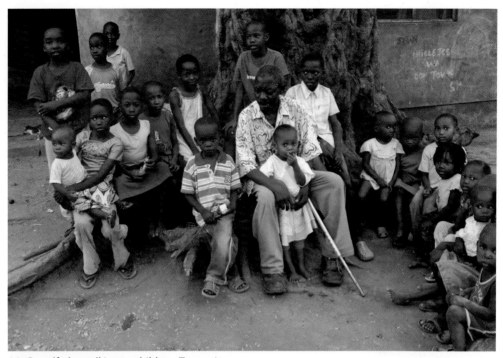

16 Grandfather talking to children, Tanzania

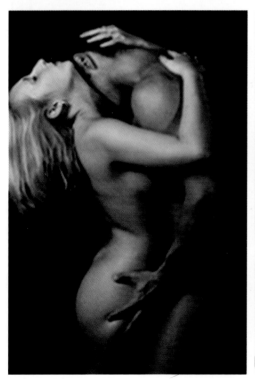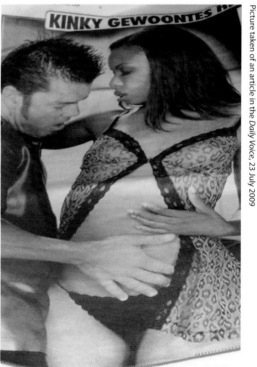

Picture taken of an article in the *Daily Voice*, 23 July 2009

17, 18 Examples of sexually explicit cellphone and newspaper images submitted by children in South Africa

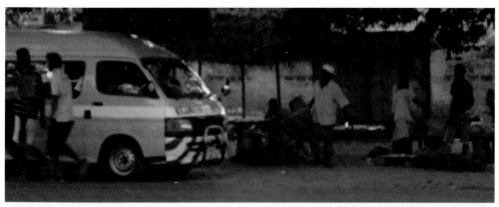

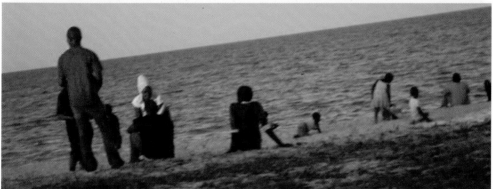

19, 20 Children witnessed sex on public transport (Tanzania) and at the beach (Kenya)

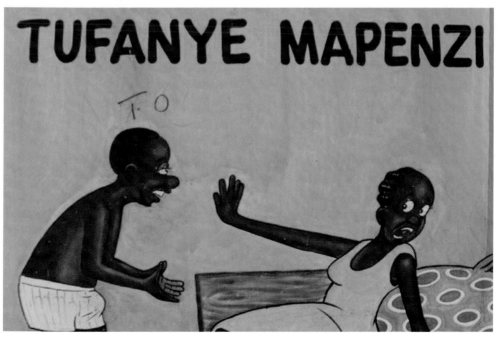

21 Billboard, Tanzania: 'No condom, no sex!'

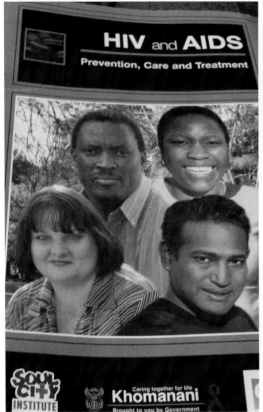

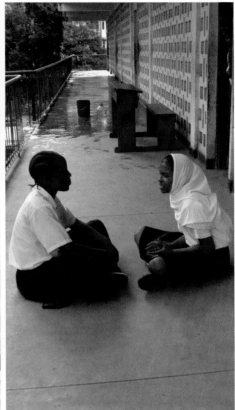

22 South African HIV/AIDS awareness campaign

23 Informal peer education in process, Tanzania

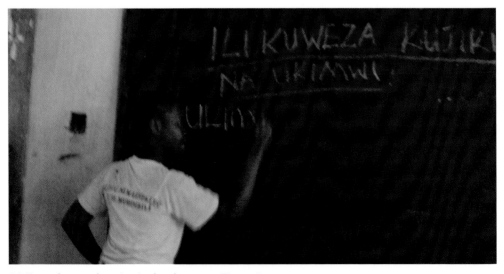

24 Formal peer education in the classroom, Tanzania

HIV/AIDS, sub-Saharan Africa and education

Questions have long been asked about children and sex education: what do they know? What do they need to know? What is the best way to teach them? Who should teach them? And how did the advent of HIV and AIDS change some of the answers to these questions? This book is a study of children's sexual knowledge and its interaction with formal schooling and local community contexts. The enquiry was undertaken in three African countries – Kenya, Tanzania and South Africa. This chapter provides the background to and overall framework for the research study.

AIDS in sub-Saharan Africa

It is over 30 years since cases of AIDS were first reported in sub-Saharan Africa. Since then much has happened. In its latest update on the epidemic, UNAIDS/WHO (2010) asserts that the spread of AIDS peaked in 1996, when 3.5 million new infections occurred. This report shows that 'the world has turned the corner – it has halted and begun to reverse the spread of HIV' (UNAIDS/WHO 2010: 7). New infections are declining in 33 countries, 22 of which are in sub-Saharan Africa. This is due to 'the impact of HIV prevention efforts plus the natural course of HIV epidemics' (UNAIDS/WHO 2010: 16). The incidence of HIV infection fell by more than 25 per cent in these 22 countries. The trend is most apparent among young people. 'The sharpest declines have showed a significant decline in HIV prevalence among young men or women in national surveys' (UNAIDS/WHO 2010: 19). In the three countries in this present study, rates either fell or stabilised between 2001 and 2009. The prevalence in Kenya fell from about 14 per cent in the mid-1990s to 5 per cent in 2006; Tanzania's rates have slowed to about 3.4 per 1 000 persons; South Africa's annual incidence among 18-year-olds declined from 1.8 per cent in 2005 to 0.8 per cent in 2008. Despite these falling rates, in South Africa the prevalence of the epidemic remains the largest in the world, and about 40 per cent of all adult women with HIV live in southern Africa (UNAIDS/WHO 2010: 28).

Sub-Saharan Africa is more severely affected by HIV/AIDS than any other region in the world. It is estimated that 1.3 million people died of HIV-related illnesses in sub-Saharan Africa in 2009, or 72 per cent of the global total of 1.8 million (UNAIDS/WHO 2010). Of all people living with HIV in 2009, 34 per cent resided in the 10 countries comprising southern Africa and 31 per cent of all new HIV infections occurred in these same countries, as did 33 per cent of all AIDS-related deaths (UNAIDS/WHO 2010: 28). Many new infections were among young people aged 15 and over, although there was a reduction in new infections among children younger than 15. In 2009 there were 32 per cent fewer newly infected children and 26 per cent fewer AIDS-related deaths among children in 2009 compared with 2004 (UNAIDS/WHO 2010: 29). To date it is estimated that 14 million children have been orphaned in sub-Saharan Africa. This is a large-scale human tragedy with children and young people at the centre of it.

The risk of becoming infected is especially disproportionate for girls and young women. UNAIDS/WHO (2010) reports that slightly more than half of all people living with HIV are women and girls. In sub-Saharan Africa, more women than men are living with HIV, and young women aged 15–24 are as much as eight times more likely than men to be HIV-positive. These rates are linked to gender-based violence and women's economic dependence on older men. In Kenya, young women between 15 and 19 are three times more likely than males to be infected, while 20- to 24-year-old women are 5.5 times more likely to be living with HIV than men in the same age cohort (KNACC 2009). Among people aged 15 to 24 in Tanzania, females are four times more likely than males to be living with HIV (Tanzanian Commission for AIDS 2008). The high prevalence of intergenerational sexual partnerships may also play an important role in young women's disproportionate risk of HIV infection (Leclerc-Madlala 2008).

Heterosexual intercourse remains the primary mode of HIV transmission in sub-Saharan Africa, with extensive ongoing transmission to newborns and breastfed babies (Leclerc-Madlala 2008.) In a number of African countries, there is evidence of increasing transmission of the virus through needle sharing among drug users and among men who have sex with men (UNAIDS/WHO 2010). These recent data show that AIDS remains a major health priority, that there is geographic variation between and within countries, that it is an evolving epidemic, that there is evidence of success in HIV prevention and that improved treatment is having an impact.

There has been much progress both in preventative efforts and in treatment programmes. Behaviour, especially that of young people, has begun to change and behaviour change is the most important factor accounting for the recent declines in new HIV infections: 'Amongst young people in 15 of the most severely affected countries, HIV prevalence has fallen by more than 25 percent as these young people have adopted safer sexual practices.' Such practices include condom use, a reduction in engaging in sexual activity with multiple partners and delaying the onset of sexual activity (UNAIDS/WHO 2010: 9). Condom availability has increased in places of need and since 'correct and consistent condom use has been found to be greater than 90 percent effective in preventing transmission of HIV and other sexually transmitted infections', this is significant progress (UNAIDS/WHO 2010: 64). The combination of preventive efforts is having an impact and is important. In Namibia, for example, improvements across key knowledge and behaviour indicators, such as comprehensive knowledge, age of sexual engagement in higher-risk sex and condom use among male and females aged 15 to 24, have been linked to declines in HIV prevalence among young people from more than 10 per cent in 2007 to 5 per cent in 2009 (UNAIDS/WHO 2010: 65).

An interesting element, and one that is important for this study, is knowledge. Comprehensive and correct knowledge about HIV has increased slightly since 2003, but at 34 per cent the number of young people with sufficient knowledge is only a third of the target of 95 per cent. Ten countries in the world have achieved 60 per cent, but Namibia is the only southern African country to have done so. All three countries in our study are among those countries where less than half of young people can correctly answer five basic questions about HIV and its transmission (UNAIDS/WHO 2010: 68). Knowledge about HIV is important and a central feature of educational interventions.

The role of education

There are two main aspects that are considered here: the general role of schooling and the specific role of HIV prevention education. The impact of HIV upon those in education is also referred to in this section.

Education in general and specific HIV-related education for young people both in and out of school are seen as among the primary means for prevention in the absence of a cure or vaccine. Recent research has shown that education is having an impact in reducing the number of new infections and that the role of formal schooling is increasingly being shown to prevent HIV (Acedo 2009; UNAIDS/WHO 2010). However, HIV/AIDS is Janus-faced: it impacts upon those in education and those in education have at the same time to turn their faces to engage in preventative work. The syndrome is a major problem for both young people and teachers in sub-Saharan African countries (Bennell et al. 2002). Young people are particularly vulnerable, and those living in poverty even more so. Teachers and teacher trainees are also vulnerable to HIV/AIDS and the pandemic has had a big impact on the teacher workforce. Teacher mortality rates are rising and Acedo (2009) notes that teachers are dying faster than they can be replaced. Schools are increasingly facing the challenge of dealing with young people who have been orphaned and whose families have been affected by HIV. High school dropout rates and low enrolment rates are especially prevalent among children who have lost one or both parents to HIV/AIDS.

Education in general

Formal education, or schooling, appears to play a protective role with regard to HIV. Bennell et al. (2002, citing Gregson et al. 2001) highlight an interesting study in Zimbabwe that showed that HIV prevalence rates were much lower among 15- to 19-year-olds who were attending school than those who were not. This is especially important for girls, since rates of infection among teenage girls are five times higher than those among boys (Baker et al. 2009). Initially, however, research showed that education was in reality a risk factor and not a protective factor – contrary to the positive relationship between increased education and improved health-related behaviours. Baker et al. give a vivid account of the slowness of sub-Saharan countries to respond to the onset of HIV. It was in 1981 that HIV was first identified in the US, and it was not until the late 1980s that it was recognised as present and problematic in African countries. In these early stages, studies noted that the virus was more prevalent among the wealthy and more educated. This was due to increased mobility and wealth. Educated men especially, were frequently more socially and sexually active. They had greater leisure time than others, more time for sexual relationships, and greater status given their wealth and leisure. Baker et al. (2009) show that this conception of education as a risk factor for HIV infection has changed over the past decade and that education is now firmly seen to be a protective factor and hence deserving of its label as a 'social vaccine' (see also Kelly 2000; World Bank 2003). There is now a wealth of evidence to show that formal education 'has a social vaccine effect even after controlling for confounding factors such as relative social status and wealth, and access to health care' (Baker et al. 2009: 473). Education, conclude Mirowski and Ross (2003), has an 'enduring, consistent and growing effect on health'. Therefore, in general, education is very powerful in helping to reduce rates of HIV, although we are not necessarily sure of the nature of the relationship, with information and knowledge transfer not being seen as a complete explanation (Baker et al. 2009). Baker et al. (2009: 481) conclude that 'there is growing evidence that resulting enhanced everyday reasoning and decision-making skills lead to healthier behaviour and avoidance of unhealthy behaviour'. However, more work needs to be done to fully understand the relationship between formal schooling and rates of HIV infection.

HIV prevention education: Policy and practice

Although HIV prevention education has become widely known as the 'social vaccine', educational responses in sub-Saharan Africa have not been speedy. This has been due to the initial conception that HIV is a condition contracted by homosexual men, the long latency period of the infection, embedded practices of transactional sex and the reluctance to act shown by a number of African governments. For example, in Kenya an effective national response was not adopted until 2000, and in South Africa, Thabo Mbeki's support of scientists who denied the existence of the virus was infamous. Some countries were quicker to respond, however, and currently all of the countries in this study and many other sub-Saharan countries have adopted HIV-related preventative education programmes and have national policies in place. These national efforts included preventative programmes in formal schooling, as well as community education programmes (Kirby 2008). Uganda was the first country in the region to run a campaign to reduce its HIV/AIDS prevalence, and has been extraordinarily successful in reducing rates from 18 per cent in 1992 to 6 per cent in 2002 (Uganda AIDS Commission 2008).

Targeted HIV prevention programmes are also having an impact on sexual behaviours in some African countries. In southern Africa, a trend towards safer sexual behaviour was observed among both young men and young women (15- to 24-year-olds) between 2000 and 2007 (Gouws et al. 2008). Shisana et al. (2009) reported a decline in new infections among teenagers aged 15 to 19 in South Africa and an increase in the proportion of adults (including teenage males) reporting condom use during their most recent episode of sexual intercourse (from 31.3 per cent in 2002 to 64.8 per cent in 2008). Nevertheless, condom use remains low in many parts of sub-Saharan Africa (Shisana et al. 2009). The latest UNAIDS/WHO (2010) update on the epidemic has confirmed this trend, namely that young people are adopting safer sexual practices, including increased usage of condoms. Therefore, this report argues that prevention programmes are having an impact among young people. A more detailed picture of HIV and AIDS prevalence rates and policies in each of the three countries that are the focus of this book is provided in Chapter 3.

However, education for HIV prevention and education in the context of high AIDS prevalence are highly challenging endeavours. Education as a central response to this medical condition comes at a price. As early as 2002, the World Bank (2002) estimated that HIV/AIDS would add between $450 and $550 million to the cost of achieving the Education For All goals in 33 African countries. In addition to this financial cost, teaching on HIV-related matters is highly contentious and problematic both for teachers and teacher educators (Mugimu & Nabadda 2009; Oluga et al. 2010). Following the initial educational response, there is now an acceptance that much more nuanced, contextual research and understanding is needed.

The nature of the response

Governments have responded to the HIV/AIDS crisis by introducing HIV-related educational programmes. The initial response to the recognised need for action was to introduce a range of programmes, including life skills, sex education, reproductive health programmes and other health interventions in schools (Aikman et al. 2008). The introduction of sexuality education in schools is justified and has been confirmed by recent trends in the decline of infection as well as by research on sex education. For example, Kirby et al. (2007) reviewed 83 studies that measured the impact of curriculum-based sex and HIV education programmes on sexual behaviour, and mediating factors among youth under 25 worldwide. Two-thirds of the programmes significantly improved one or more sexual behaviours. The evidence is strong that programmes do not hasten or increase sexual behaviour but, instead, that some programmes delay or decrease sexual behaviours or increase condom or contraceptive use.

The management and implementation of such programmes is complex and there are different degrees of progress and success. For example, Coombe and Kelly (2002) report that many programmes lacked connections to the social pressures experienced by young people or to their decision-making and social experiences. Other researchers have argued strongly for the need to understand more about how young people contextualise their knowledge (Allen 2005; Brown et al. 2001). Although there have been evaluations of young people's knowledge about HIV/AIDS, there is a need for in-depth, small-scale qualitative studies that focus on 'the perspectives and experiences of youth in different settings' (Brown et al. 2001: 46). This way, we will gain a better understanding of the social dynamics that contribute to the impact and conduct of sexuality education in schools (Campbell et al. 2005; Esat. 2003).

Approaches are not necessarily driven by evidence-based understandings. For example, Boler and Aggleton (2005) critique the introduction of life skills into school curricula and suggest there is a lack of evidence regarding its effectiveness, despite being adopted by UN programmes and national educational ministries. They identify two key approaches to HIV prevention education. One set of approaches is underpinned by the belief that individuals have substantial control over their actions, an approach followed by a group of academics whom they label as rationalists, or bounded rationalists. The other group, the structuralists, view human action as 'influenced more by underlying economic, social and cultural structures' (Boler & Aggleton 2005: 1). Although these characterisations are polarised, they argue that most attempts to date have been in the rationalist camp, with an emphasis on rational choice and individual agency. This present study leans towards a structuralist approach to prevention education, with the emphasis on social context and structure. A fuller exploration of HIV-related education and sex education is undertaken in Chapter 3. However, as can be seen from this discussion, there is much debate to be had about the nature of HIV-related education and much research is still needed.

This project and its aims

The theoretical frameworks that this study employs are the sociocultural influences on HIV-related education in schools (Campbell 2003), consulting pupils for school improvement (Rudduck & McIntyre 2007), and Basil Bernstein's (1999) distinction between informal, everyday knowledge and formal, in-school knowledge. These frameworks also inform our use of the term 'knowledges', rather than only 'knowledge', to highlight the social context that informs how young people come to know what they know, rather than placing emphasis only on what they know. This section expands on these frameworks. They re-emerge and are further discussed throughout our analysis.

We know that young people are particularly at risk of HIV infection for a multiplicity of reasons, including youthful experimentation and risk taking in developing adult and sexual identity, and a lack of understanding of their vulnerability. This is exacerbated by poverty (Rivers & Aggleton 1999), a key feature of the three countries in which our study is conducted. De Waal (2002: 171) argues that HIV/AIDS is the 'single greatest threat facing Africa's young people today'. As has already been said, research into schooling and HIV is still in its infancy and efforts have focused largely on the evaluation of educational interventions in terms of behaviour change, with knowledge, attitude, belief practices and intentions of target audiences of such interventions being measured. Many have argued that the sort of educational programmes in existence do not meet the needs of young people and do not take sufficient account of the sociocultural aspects of their lives (Allen 2007; Campbell 2003). Some research has shown the importance of sociocultural, political and economic influences on the vulnerability of young people to HIV/AIDS (Campbell et al. 2005; Esat 2003; Rivers & Aggleton 1999). However, this is not yet sufficient to inform practice. Consequently, the first important idea in this study was to take into account the sociocultural context and processes that surround HIV-related education in schools.

The second important concept is that of consulting pupils. There has been a focus on consulting pupils about their education in the last decade and this has been linked to notions of rights and voice (Arnot et al. 2004; Nieto 1994; Rudduck & Flutter 2000). The United Nations Convention on the Rights of the Child has largely driven this agenda. There has also begun to be both consultation with young people about matters of sexuality and HIV/AIDS-related education and arguments for it (Allen 2007; Bhana 2007a; Campbell 2003; Pattman & Chege 2003). The practice of consulting pupils about their classroom experience is complex and challenging but highly profitable, in terms of what can be learnt about practices and perceptions (Rudduck & McIntyre 2007). There is a need to interrogate young people's experiences and views on sex and AIDS-related education much more, and this has also been a key driver of this study

However, the work of educational theorist Basil Bernstein drove us to go further than consultation. In thinking about schooling and the curriculum, Bernstein (1999) distinguished between horizontal and vertical knowledges and discourses. The horizontal is seen as everyday, oral, common-sense discourse, which has a group of features: local, segmental, context-dependent, tacit, multilayered, and often contradictory across contexts but not within contexts. Horizontal discourse is normally acquired from peers and significant others in the young person's immediate context. The vertical is the formal discourse of schooling: codified, assessed and authoritative. We wanted to understand both of these and to explore the possibility of crossing these borders and of breaking these hard educational boundaries. We aimed to establish young people's views on the ways in which sex and AIDS education is conducted, and how pedagogies and curricula on offer interact with their own social, cultural and individual contexts. Therefore, this study aimed to examine young people's varying sexual knowledges and to go further by exploring how they are used and interact with AIDS education programmes in school.

We set ourselves two main research questions. The first asked where do children get their information about sex and AIDS and what do they know about these topics? We were especially eager to find out whether and in what way this information differs depending on where it was learnt. The second question asks how this informal information interacts with the formal sex and AIDS education received in the classroom. This second question was crucial to our overall research aim of finding out how young people's sexual knowledges might be used to effect change in pedagogy and the curriculum.

We were, therefore, interested in teachers' understandings and awareness of young people's contexts and sexual knowledges, as well as the interactions during AIDS education in the classroom. The socio-cultural aims that we believed to be crucial necessitated exploring community members' views too. There have been some recent attempts to survey young people's sources of knowledge (Bennell et al. 2002), but this has not received a detailed examination. We know little about the nature, sources and processes of the knowledges that young people bring into the classroom. Nor do we know how these knowledges are acquired, the importance young people attach to them, the ways in which poverty produces specific knowledges, or the way in which these knowledges interact with extant curricula and pedagogies.

In this study we begin to answer these questions. At the same time, we are already able to see how these understandings can be used to develop hybrid curricula – collaborations between teachers and pupils that 'bridg[e]…school knowledge or public knowledge and the students' own cultural knowledge, and thus encourag[e] students to analyse this interaction and then use the knowledge learned to take charge of their lives' (Taylor 2000: 58). Therefore, this monograph highlights children's sexual knowledges in three African countries, Tanzania, Kenya and South Africa, and explores the potential for a hybrid project with regard to sex and AIDS education among primary-aged children. Chapter 2 describes in some detail how we went about consulting children and key stakeholders' voices through a multi-year research-and-development process.

CHAPTER 2

Consulting children and stakeholders through research

In this study we examined children's views on how AIDS education programmes in school were and should be conducted. Teachers' understandings and awareness of young people's contexts and sexual knowledges were also examined, as were community stakeholders. We were also interested to understand the barriers to teachers' use of community-based knowledge in their practice, with a view to enhancing the delivery of AIDS education in classrooms in the developing world. In this chapter we detail our research questions, the approach that we adopted to answer these and our methodological learnings while in the field. We conclude with a reflection on the ethical issues encountered in researching with children and in the context of cultural sensibilities around sex education. This chapter also provides details of our research tools, available in full in Appendix 1.

Aims and design of the study

This study, which comprises a sample of eight schools in three countries in sub-Saharan Africa – Kenya, South Africa and Tanzania – aims to examine the sources, contents and processes of children's community-based sexual knowledges, and asks how these knowledges interact with AIDS education programmes in school. It takes a step back from 'what works' in the classroom in terms of sex and HIV/AIDS education, and asks two fundamental intellectual questions, which have considerable implications for practice:

- What are the primary sources and contents of sexual knowledges for young people in sub-Saharan Africa, and how do these knowledges differ in terms of content and process of acquisition?
- How do these knowledges interact with AIDS education received in the classroom, and how might young people's sexual knowledges be used to effect change in pedagogy and the curriculum?

These questions were investigated using multiple research methods over the course of two years of research and development in eight schools (three in Kenya, three in Tanzania and two in South Africa). All three countries, although somewhat different in their levels and distribution of poverty, have relatively high HIV infection levels, and have marked interplays between Christian, Islamic and traditional practices. We chose the schools in each country as important case studies, which we expected would provide significant transferable insights into sex and AIDS education in a number of developing countries.

Through a variety of innovative research methods to elicit data, including digital still photography and mini-video documentaries, as well as interviews and observations, primary-aged children and key stakeholders were asked to discuss what children knew about sex education and AIDS, how they came to know and how their formal and informal sexual knowledges interacted in the classroom. To explore the interaction between the knowledges that children bring into the classroom (i.e. everyday knowledges) and the formal messages disseminated by teachers and policy-makers (i.e. institutional knowledges) it was necessary to study the school setting and teachers' understandings and aware-ness of young people's contexts, as well as the interactions during AIDS and sex-education lessons in the classroom. The methods were designed to engage as fully as possible with the underlying issues, difficulties and dilemmas faced by teachers as agents of sexual knowledge, and to learn about schools as spaces of sexual knowledge. These methods took every opportunity to document the discourses and social interactions that permeate social, cultural and religious worlds, and ultimately offer ways in which these knowledges can be integrated into formative AIDS education.

The study proceeded in six stages, summarised in Table 2.1. Stage I involved a 'rapid ethnography' (discussed in more detail later in the chapter), whose purpose was to understand the school context, including socio-economic levels, the relationship between pupils and teachers, the overall school cli-mate and the pedagogy and challenges faced by each school. The rapid ethnography also included observations of HIV/AIDS and sex-education classes, and offered opportunities to get to know pupils and teachers and build the rapport necessary for an ongoing research project.

Stage II was the main data-collection process of ascertaining pupils', teachers' and community stakehold-ers' perceptions of current sex-education practices and children's needs. Methods included sources of sexual knowledge photovoice activities, individual interviews and focus group discussions (FGDs) with pupils, as well as current and desired sex-education mini-documentaries. Initial interviews related to the photovoice activity, and asked children to talk about where they obtained their knowledge about sex, love, relationships and HIV/AIDS; second interviews focused on questions relating to gender, religion and culture difference in sex education. With teachers and community stakeholders, individual interviews and FGDs were held, using the desired sex-education mini-documentaries as discussion starters with both groups, in addition to asking wider questions of both groups about content and pedagogy.

Stage III comprised face-to-face meetings among the researchers following an intensive period of the-matic data coding in order to share results across all three countries and find common themes from the data. There were two such meetings – one in Cambridge and the other in Dar es Salaam. The second meeting also produced an outline for the community dialogues which formed Stage IV.

Stage IV, which consisted of community dialogues, provided an opportunity to report back to study participants and key stakeholders on findings at that point. In addition, it provided an opportunity to ensure that this research study was collaborative and that those who would implement its findings were integrally involved in the study. The questions that guided these community dialogues are also available in Appendix 1. Key to these dialogues was the need for pupils to feel free to speak their minds even in the presence of adults. This was achieved by laying down clear ground rules before the discus-sion, creating an atmosphere conducive to friendly discussion, and perspective taking (i.e. inviting participants to see a dilemma from the point of view of the other party). For example, teachers were asked to consider parents' points of views, pupils to consider teachers' points of views and religious leaders to consider children's needs.

Stage V collated findings and methods into a toolkit for consulting pupils about sex education in African contexts in the school environment. The aim of the toolkit was to provide guidelines so that teachers responsible for sex and AIDS education might develop a local 'hybrid curriculum' (Bernstein 1996). It is not a curriculum in itself, but offers activities and theoretical guidelines for enhancing cur-rent syllabi in order to incorporate children's everyday knowledges into the institutional knowledge presupposed by the official curriculum. Appendix 2 provides the toolkit in written form; a visual format that includes links to videos, photographs and source documents is also available on a dedicated web-site – www.educ.cam.ac.uk/centres/cce/askaids.

TABLE 2.1 *Six stages of the research process*

Stage	Activity	Description
I	Rapid ethnography	Sketches of each school context, including socio-economic levels, relationships between pupils and teachers, school climate, pedagogy and general challenges faced by each school.
II	Data collection	Methods included photovoice on sources of sexual knowledge, mini-video documentaries on current and desired sex education, and interviews and FGDs with pupils, teachers and community stakeholders.
III	Analysis	Analysis done in each country and in face-to-face meetings of researchers; included sources of pupils' sexuality, dilemmas in teaching sex education, communities' views on sex education, and sex education pedagogies in use and desired by pupils.
IV	Community dialogues	These were used to provide feedback to study participants and elicit further data, as stakeholders commented on data already presented and were encouraged to see dilemmas from each other's points of view.
V	Toolkit development	Data obtained from the study was used to help teachers implement a hybrid sex-education curriculum in the classroom.
VI	Implementation pilot	Interactively work with and support schools and community stakeholders to test the toolkit as a vehicle for consulting children on sex education and developing a hybrid curriculum.

Stage VI is the implementation pilot and will not be reported on in this monograph. However, we will describe how we envisage that the toolkit will be used in classrooms and our hopes for how it could materially change the ways in which sex and AIDS education is conducted among children in Africa.

Beginning the study – Ethics, sampling and access

In each country we followed the same protocol of obtaining ethical clearance, choosing schools, negotiating access and selecting participants. The following sections provide details for each of these processes and document the challenges encountered in each country.

Obtaining ethical clearance

Formal ethical clearance for the project was obtained from the Research Ethics Committee of the Human Sciences Research Council (HSRC) in South Africa. This ethics committee is nationally accredited by the South African government. In the absence of formal ethics committees in Kenya and Tanzania, ethical clearance was obtained from the Aga Khan University Institute of Education, which operates in both Tanzania and Kenya. We ensured that the three canons of research ethics were closely followed, namely confidentiality, child protection and informed consent. With regard to confidentiality, all names used in this monograph are pseudonyms. In particular, since visual materials are an important part of this study, care has been taken to safeguard the identities of individuals in still and video images. With regard to the use of visual portrayals of third parties, we only used images where they do not prejudice the research participant or the person portrayed. In addition, all data transcribers signed a confidentiality agreement stating that they would not discuss the data with anyone.

From the point of view of child protection, we made referral sources available to children should they need to speak to a counsellor about upsetting issues, especially in relation to ongoing sexual abuse or violence.

With regard to informed consent, all child participants and their de facto caregivers were asked for assent and consent, respectively. Information sheets were explained to children (in the language of their own choosing) with a written supporting document. Parents were asked for permission for their children's participation, while children were asked to agree to participate. All adult participants, such as teachers and community stakeholders, were asked for written consent. Appendix 3 provides copies of the informed consent forms for children and adults.

Choosing schools

In choosing sites we were particularly interested in ensuring that schools were representative of every-day schools in each country, that there would be a mix of boys and girls, and children from diverse religious and cultural backgrounds. In Kenya this meant that Mombasa would be the best site to ensure a mix of children from Christian, Muslim and strongly traditional households all in one district. In Tanzania, this was easily achieved in and around Dar es Salaam. In South Africa, Cape Town offered cultural and religious diversity, as well as some racial[1] diversity, with South Africa's School A comprising black children and School B comprising coloured children.

Schools were purposively selected because we were interested in understanding how religion and culture, especially cultural restrictions and taboos, impact on children's acquisition of sexual knowledges. Dar es Salaam, Mombasa and Cape Town are all port cities and tourist hubs, and consequently all three sites are fairly cosmopolitan. Each of these cities' communities are vulnerable to HIV/AIDS infection, and they are major sites for intervention. The existence of tourism alongside high levels of poverty, and the mobility of workers in the transport and shipping industries have engendered the growth of female and male prostitution, and intergenerational sex. Children were aware of these features of their cities, and we both expected and discovered that children's exposure to sexual knowledge was high.

Negotiating access

In all three countries, access to schools began with the applications for permission to conduct research through the Ministry of Education (in Tanzania and Kenya) or local Department of Basic Education (South Africa). In Kenya a research permit was obtained from the national ministry in Nairobi upon submission of letters of support from the Cambridge Centre for Commonwealth Education and the Aga Khan Institute of Education. Once obtained, the permit was presented to the district education officer in Mombasa District, who, in turn, introduced the researcher to the Municipal Education Office, where the researcher presented a copy of the research permit. The Municipal Education Office then worked with the researcher to select three schools based on our stated criteria of gender, religious and cultural diversity, as well as some diversity between urban and rural areas. We ended up with one rural and two urban primary schools. The urban schools were set in dissimilar environments: one had children drawn predominantly from a nearby slum and the other had a mixture of children from different social classes – but most of whom were poor. In Tanzania, the process of access was similar,

---

1   Racial terminology is problematic in South Africa. We reluctantly follow the legacy of the Apartheid system of racial classification, as defined by the South African Population Registration Act of 1950, for descriptive purposes – 'black', 'white', 'coloured' and 'Indian'. Currently in South Africa, it remains standard practice to use these (or other) descriptors in order to call attention to continuing inequalities and their effects. Some use 'African' or 'black African' instead of 'black', whereas some capitalise both terms; yet others use 'black' to include people described as 'coloured'. Our use of these terms is pragmatic and does not imply endorsement of these classifications.

with permission being sought from the National and District Ministries of Education. There were some delays in obtaining permission to research in schools because separate ministries dealt with education and non-governmental organisations' (NGO) involvement in schools, and the Aga Khan University was considered an NGO. Ultimately, seven schools were selected by the ministry, but the researchers narrowed these down to three (two rural, one urban) after visiting the schools and being refused permission by some. In South Africa, negotiating access was somewhat simpler. The provincial Department of Education required the research protocol to be submitted, including research instruments and a list of schools from which the participating schools would be chosen. A letter of permission was then issued and supplied to the school head after he or she had agreed to participate in the study. One school declined participation due to 'busy-ness'. Both schools were peri-urban, although School A included a number of pupils who had recently migrated from a rural area.

Table 2.2 provides a brief sketch of each of the eight schools in this study. A more comprehensive portrait of each school, along with an analytical comparison of schools in all three counties, is provided in Chapter 4, while Chapter 3 provides an overall educational and HIV policy overview of each of the three countries.

TABLE 2.2 *Thumbnail sketch of participating schools*

Kenya School A

Kenya School A is a rural school 20 km from the main Mombasa–Malindi highway. At the time of the study, it had a total of 12 teachers (2 female, 10 male), 728 primary pupils (342 boys, 386 girls) and 117 children in kindergarten. The access road to the school was via a long, winding dirt road in a sparsely populated, very dry, and clearly impoverished area. Nearby was the city's rubbish dump site. Despite its environment, the school had a strong ethos of learning, with pupils working on their own even when teachers were absent. The school had a feeding programme that had increased the enrolment rate. Most of the children came from families who lived in nearby shacks or squatter areas. Economic activities included small-scale farming, cattle herding and selling *mnazi* (coconut brew) and water.

Kenya School B

Kenya School B is located in Mombasa. It had a total of 13 teachers (3 male, 10 female) and 450 pupils. Of these, 50 had been identified as orphaned and vulnerable children, 10 of whom were HIV-positive. Its catchment area was a mixture of informal settlements, and lower-class and upmarket housing. The pupil population, however, originated mostly from the informal settlements. This school had an active HIV/AIDS club because one of the teachers was well trained in HIV/AIDS education. Many parents were single parents or divorced and many children lived with their grandmothers. They had a school feeding programme, with well-wishers donating fruit and vegetables to the 50 orphaned and vulnerable children. Of the three Kenyan schools, this was dirtiest, with littered classrooms and grounds.

Kenya School C

Kenya School C is located in downtown Mombasa off a busy road. It had a total of 17 teachers (5 male, 12 female) and 477 pupils (247 boys, 230 girls). Its catchment area was a mixture of informal settlements and lower- and middle-class housing. It had a kindergarten, special education unit and an active feeding programme. The head teacher said that approximately 300 of the children ate the free food, while the rest brought their own packed lunch. Unlike the two other Kenyan schools, this one had a larger population of children from lower-middle-class families, although 90 per cent of the pupils were from slums. It also had a smaller class population of 25–30 pupils per class. The school had an HIV/AIDS club called 'Chill' (meaning abstain/wait). The school looked very well kept, had toys and a playground for the kindergarten children.

→

Tanzania School A

Tanzania school A is located in an economically disadvantaged ward of Kinondoni Municipality. The school had 33 teachers (7 males, 26 females) and 1 073 pupils (512 males and 561 females). Of these, three were known to be HIV-positive. It is poorly resourced, with few desks and poor ventilation in classrooms. The class sizes range from 65 to 76 pupils. The school is close to an area well known for sex work and substance abuse. Its catchment area is a mixture of slums and lower- and middle-class houses. Most pupils live with their parents in rented houses and are of low economic status. The majority of the parents are self-employed, working as petty traders, food vendors, watchmen and domestic workers.

Tanzania School B

Tanzania school B is a government school that serves a lower-middle-class population. It is situated in a large compound with three buildings, and shares these buildings, the school compound and adjacent football ground with another school. Children in the school are from mixed backgrounds. Those pupils from educated and well-off families either use buses provided by the school or are dropped off by parents, whereas many poorer children are known to walk for over an hour to get to school. Some affluent parents provide financial support to students who need it. The teacher:pupil ratio is 1:26, which is atypical, but this is calculated from the number of teachers registered. In reality, however, there are fewer teachers at school owing to study leave, sick leave and maternity leave, which makes the ratio closer to 1:40. There are known cases of HIV/AIDS in this school, although the school administration is not aware of the exact numbers.

Tanzania School C

Tanzania school C is in a poor locality that is home to a mixture of Muslims, Christians and those adhering to traditional religions. It is about 15 km from the city centre and served by a local ferry crossing. Pupils come from the neighbouring areas. The student population was 615, with an equal number of boys and girls. Female teachers outnumber male teachers. The teacher:student ratio is 1:43. There is a water project in the neighbourhood provided by an NGO that is also the source of employment for a number of parents. Pupils at this school are frequently barefooted. The school has no running water, which means no drinking water. There is a separate teacher for health education.

South Africa School A

South Africa School A is in a peri-urban black township approximately 11 km from the city of Cape Town. It is one of 11 primary schools in the township and is ranked by the local educational authorities as a quintile 3 school (schools are ranked by resources and poverty level – 1 is lowest, 5 is highest). Its language of instruction is isiXhosa and its teacher:pupil ratio is 1:42. A fee-paying school, it charges annual fees of R200. The school is well resourced and has brightly painted classrooms, a feeding scheme and playing fields. Most of the children who attend walk to school from a nearby informal settlement (slum). Neighbourhood children who can afford it, cross over the nearby highway and attend a better-quality school in the adjacent coloured community.

South Africa School B

South Africa School B is located in what was demarcated a coloured area during Apartheid. Approximately 10 km from Cape Town, it has more and less impoverished catchment areas. The school is located in a poorer part of the community that is infamous for social problems, including substance abuse, organised gangsterism, crime and early parenting. The school is currently ranked as a quintile 5 school, but this belies its current context. It charges annual school fees of R500, and the medium of instruction is English. It has a teacher:pupil ratio of 1:38.

Table 2.3 provides a comparison of the eight schools by religious affiliation of pupils, location, teacher-to-pupil ratio and school fees.

TABLE 2.3 *Comparison of key features of participating schools*

School	Location	Religious composition	Teacher: pupil ratio	Instruction medium	School fees
Kenya School A	Rural	Muslims: 50% Christians: 50%	1 : 61	English	None, but Ksh150 per month expected for fuel and cooks' wages. Books, stationery and uniform are additional.
Kenya School B	City centre	Muslims: 70% Christians: 30%	1 : 35	English	None, but Ksh150 per month expected for fuel and cooks' wages. Books, stationery and uniform are additional.
Kenya School C	City centre	Muslims: 60% Christians: 40%	1 : 28	English	None, but Ksh150 per month expected for fuel and cooks' wages. Books, stationery and uniform are additional.
Tanzania School A	Semi-urban	Muslims: 75% Christians: 25%	1 : 32	Kiswahili	None, but school charges Tsh20 000 for desk and uniform.
Tanzania School B	City centre	Muslims: 50% Christians: 50%	1 : 26	Kiswahili	None, but school charges Tsh6 600 for uniform.
Tanzania School C	Semi-urban	Muslims: 65% Christians: 35%	1 : 43	Kiswahili	None, but school charges Tsh500 for uniform logo.
South Africa School A	Peri-urban township	100% Christian	1 : 42	isiXhosa	R200 plus uniform
South Africa School B	Coloured area	Muslims: 50% Christians: 50%	1 : 38	English	R500 plus uniform

Selecting participants

Selecting participants turned out to be far more challenging than expected. Since this was a qualitative study, we were relying on a purposive sample and needed approximately 15 to 20 children to participate in each school. However, individual classes were frequently far larger than these numbers and so selection criteria had to be employed.

In South Africa, in both schools there were approximately 40 students in the Grade 6 class. For video activities we included all children, whereas for interviews and photovoice we made our selection on the basis of, firstly, those who returned consent forms and, secondly, to satisfy our criteria of gender balance, religious-affiliation balance and some cultural diversity. We achieved this by ensuring that we obtained basic demographic data from children at the outset of the process. As we got to know the children, we also made the pragmatic decision to interview those whose ease of communication we felt would make for better interviews. In any event, we continued interviewing until saturation had been reached. In Kenya this occurred sooner than in South Africa and Tanzania. We made every effort for children not to feel left out, although not all who wanted to participate got the opportunity in equal measure in all activities. In Kenya, children were asked to choose representatives for some activities (especially the photovoice activity) in which we clearly could not include all the children in the class due to limited equipment. Teachers in all three countries also assisted in choosing children who would be asked to conduct photovoice activities. Their choice was based mainly on their knowledge of the children's home environments and their ability to safely handle a digital camera. In South Africa teachers were reluctant to allow some pupils to take photographs because they lived in 'dangerous areas' or had parents who had substance-abuse problems and who were likely to 'sell the cameras for drug money'. Overall, we received no negative feedback from children or teachers regarding children's participation. And there were no stolen cameras – a great concern of teachers – although one camera in South Africa was accidentally broken. It got stood on!

In all schools, the head teachers were involved in selecting which teachers and community stakeholders would participate. Priority was given to teachers who were involved in HIV/AIDS teaching, the guidance/counselling teacher, the class teacher, the special-education teacher and the heads themselves. In South Africa 11 teachers participated, in Kenya 19 and in Tanzania 15.

With regard to stakeholders, a number of strategies were employed. In Kenya School A, the male deputy head teacher identified and invited community stakeholders to participate, with the result that all the stakeholders chosen were men (the chairman of the school, a catechist, a Muslim elder, a village elder and the assistant to the chief). In Kenya School B, the school head requested a female village elder to be the contact person and to introduce the researcher to stakeholders. This worked well, since the researcher could ensure a balance of representatives. In School A in South Africa, the researcher, who was a resident in the community, invited local stakeholders to attend; in school B the school head invited stakeholders. In Tanzania, invitations were also somewhat gendered – with the male researcher and male teachers inviting male stakeholders and the female researcher and female teachers inviting female stakeholders.

In all, 40 community stakeholders participated in the study. There were 13 in South Africa (two parents, two grandparents, one nurse, one NGO worker, one traditional healer, two school heads, one community health worker, one community sports worker, one Muslim leader, one Christian leader); 14 in Kenya (three doctors, one HIV-positive woman, one chief's assistant, one priest, one school chairperson, two female parents, three village elders, one councillor's assistant, one youth representative); and 13 in Tanzania (five religious-education teachers, three parents, three school committee members, one traditional practitioner, one police officer). Table 2.4 summarises the numbers of research participants in the study.

In total, the study comprised 125 child participants, 45 teacher participants and 40 community stakeholders in eight schools. In addition, we observed 64 lessons, and ran eight focus groups with teachers and three with community stakeholders. Children produced 840 photographs as part of the photovoice activity and 21 mini-documentaries.

As for gender, there were nearly equal numbers of boys and girls in the study, although more female teachers than males participated. This is representative of the gender make-up of primary-school teachers in the three countries.

TABLE 2.4 *Numbers of participants and data-collection activities, by country*

	South Africa	Kenya	Tanzania	Total
Schools	2	3	3	8
Lesson observations	9	48	9	66
Child participants	38 (19 girls, 19 boys)	45 (22 girls, 23 boys)	42 (24 girls, 18 boys)	125 (65 girls, 60 boys)
Children's religious affiliation	31 Christians 7 Muslims	18 Christians 27 Muslims	15 Christians 27 Muslims	64 Christians 61 Muslims
Mini-video documentaries	4 groups	13 groups	4 groups	21 groups
Teacher participants	11 (8 female, 3 male)	19 (11 female, 8 male)	15 (9 female, 6 male)	45 (28 female, 17 male)
Stakeholders	13	14	13	40

Data-collection activities and challenges

The length of time taken to collect data differed in each country. In Kenya, data collection took place over an intensive two-month period; in South Africa it took place over a six-month period; in Tanzania data collection took nearly 10 months to complete. These varying periods of time were due to a combination of practical issues and research challenges. In Kenya the researcher was internationally based and so for practical reasons data had to be collected over a short, intensive period. In both Tanzania and South Africa researchers were locally based and research took place at the convenience of participating schools.

Earlier we have briefly described the data-collection methods and activities used; in the following sections we provide a more detailed evaluation of how each research activity worked, and the challenges encountered in implementing each activity.

Lesson observations and rapid ethnography

The first stage of data collection consisted primarily of observations. We were interested in gaining an in-depth understanding of the real situations in both the schools our participants attended and in the communities in which they resided. We also wanted to build rapport with children and teachers. Therefore, we designed two observation tools (see Appendix 1). The first consisted of a week of ethnographic observation of the schools' context – what Millen (2000) calls 'rapid ethnography' – an ethnography that employs 'time deepening strategies' and what Handwerker (2001) calls 'quick' or focused ethnography, in which specific aspects of culture, as opposed to culture in general, are the focus of research. The second was a series of lesson observations (Flanders 1970) – discussed in Chapter 6 – which were designed to highlight the types of interaction that occurred between pupil and teacher during lessons. For instance, did teachers talk most or were pupils encouraged to talk? Did teachers talk to children or at them? We wanted both to observe practice first-hand and hear what teachers, pupils and stakeholders had to say about practice.

These observations, which are fully reported in Chapter 4 (rapid ethnography) and Chapter 6 (lesson observations), added insight and depth to our data. They also provided a form of triangulation, as we were able to compare what we had seen with what we had heard. By observing the impoverished environment of their schools and homes, we were able to contextualise children's lives. In Kenya, we saw slums, mud houses and the nearby rubbish dump in which people scavenged. In South Africa, we saw the fear of crime and the dire family circumstances in which children lived. In Tanzania we observed the pervasive influence of religion through daily calls to prayer.

Photovoice

The first activity with pupils involved them taking pictures of their sources of HIV/AIDS and sexuality information. Children were asked to take photographs of the people, places and things from which they learnt about sex, love, AIDS and relationships. In Kenya teachers were asked to coordinate the activity; in South Africa and Tanzania the researchers coordinated the activity, periodically dropping off and collecting cameras, batteries and memory cards. Children got to keep the cameras for between two and seven days, after which teachers would replace the memory cards, and label and store them, or researchers would download photographs onto laptops and pass the cameras on to the next child.

To prepare pupils for the task, they were trained to use digital cameras, and given opportunities to take photographs under supervision, delete pictures and change batteries if necessary. During this training, pupils were asked to come to the front of the class, switch on the camera and take a photograph of his/her classmates. Pictures were then checked and pupils were asked to repeat the process until they were able to take good-quality photos. All participants enjoyed this training and were animated at being able to learn a new skill. Researchers also role-played with children to show them how they might approach people and ask them for permission to take their picture. This exercise allowed children to discuss how they should respond if people did not want their pictures taken or what to do if they wanted to take a sensitive picture, for example that of a brothel. Pupils came away from the training equipped to take photographs, but many immediately ran into problems – especially over concerns for their safety and that of the cameras. Many children were afraid that the cameras would be stolen and were reluctant to take them outside of their homes or schools. Although pupils were encouraged to stick to the theme, many took various pictures of themselves and their families unrelated to the study. Many ran out of batteries taking pictures of themselves with family and friends. This had the effect of lengthening the time needed to complete this assignment.

In School B in South Africa, safety was especially problematic. Children feared being robbed of cameras and were also afraid that their caregivers would take the cameras from them. Some were afraid that parents would sell the cameras to buy alcohol or drugs. Other parents were afraid they would be held financially accountable if their children lost cameras. In this school especially, children mostly took photographs of books and newspapers depicting information about AIDS and relationships. In South Africa School B, researchers had to work especially hard to encourage children to take photographs, sometimes rewarding those who completed the task in the shortest possible time (with a chocolate). In this same school, one camera was accidentally damaged (stood on), and another had a school bag stolen with a camera in it. The pupil's mother was upset and said that had the child had not taken part in the project, his school bag would not have been stolen. In South Africa School A, on one occasion the researcher accompanied pupils on a walkabout of the community in order to complete the task. In Tanzania pupils also took longer than expected to complete the project. Many deleted photographs accidentally, did not take enough pictures and were afraid to use the cameras in the community. The sporadic electricity supply also meant that it took longer than expected to charge the camera and laptop batteries, thereby extending the time needed to complete this activity.

In-depth interviews

In-depth, individual interviews were held with all participants – pupils, teachers and community stake-holders. Immediately after photovoice activities children were interviewed and asked to talk about the photographs they had taken. Key in these interviews were discussions about which sources taught them about love, sex, relationships and AIDS. In the second interview children were asked to comment on how their gender, religion and culture affected their perception of HIV/AIDS education and sexuality issues. These interview questions are provided in Appendix 1. A few challenges were encountered in interviewing children. These included the noisiness of the environment and lack of privacy, the inability of children to adequately express themselves on some of these topics and some difficulty with language. In South Africa children who were not involved in the study were naturally curious and would peer through the classroom windows to try to hear what was happening in interviews or would interrupt the interviews. Some pupils would tire of waiting for their interviews and go home – out of hunger or boredom. Researchers overcame some of these difficulties by conducting interviews in nearby homes and repeatedly rescheduling interviews.

In South Africa School B, the medium of instruction was English, although many children spoke Afrikaans as their home language. To help children express themselves better a second researcher was engaged to conduct interviews in Afrikaans. In the Kenyan context where children became embar-rassed at trying to express themselves in Swahili, especially with regard to sexual terms and acts, the researcher switched to English during interviews. Children were somehow less embarrassed to speak about sex in English.

As interviews progressed, researchers in all three countries continually compared experiences and made slight modifications to the research design. In Kenya, for example, interviews were concluded once saturation point had been reached. In South Africa the researcher asked pupils to complete an activity sheet that helped them differentiate which photographs taught them about sex, which about AIDS and which about love and relationships, since it was found that children were not differentiat-ing during interviews. This activity helped them articulate more nuanced views in later interviews. In Tanzania numerous school disruptions, including timetabling problems, unanticipated holidays, voter registration and exam marking, frequently delayed the interviews.

At the outset of the study teachers were interviewed individually and asked to reflect on effective teaching in the area of HIV and AIDS, and to talk about the barriers they experienced to effective teaching in this area. These interviews were brief and in all three countries proceeded with only a few problems. In Tanzania teachers would ask for a daily allowance for participating because this is the practice when teachers are asked to participate in workshops arranged by the Ministry of Education. Some were reluctant to participate when informed that no daily allowance was available. In Kenya, a few teachers said they did not want their interviews recorded because they were embarrassed about their ability to speak English. In South Africa teachers were frequently too busy to be interviewed, and interviews were repeatedly rescheduled. Ultimately, all the interviews were concluded and yielded important data.

Towards the conclusion of the study, short individual interviews were held with key community stake-holders. Stakeholders were asked questions about how, in their opinions, culture and religion affect AIDS education in schools. In addition, stakeholders were asked to offer their opinions on the role schools should play in educating children about AIDS, and to offer advice regarding how AIDS edu-cation ought to be delivered in schools. These interviews generally went smoothly, with only a few exceptions. In Tanzania, for example, the male researcher found it problematic to interview female community stakeholders (because of religious taboos). In addition, as we have already discussed, a male head teacher in Kenya identified only male stakeholders to be interviewed. As can be seen from the list of those who were interviewed, there was little consistency among the three countries, and even individual school sites, as to who were considered stakeholders. Parents, grandparents and religious leaders were selected in all three sites, but some sites included a policeman, while others included a traditional healer, a chief's assistant, a nurse and a community sports worker. Nevertheless, as with the teacher interviews, these stakeholders had much to contribute.

Mini-video documentaries

A key interactive activity in which pupils were asked to participate was that of making mini-video documentaries. The goal of the activity was to record children's perceptions of current AIDS-education classes, and to capture how they desired these classes to be. In groups of five, pupils were asked to prepare short 'current' and 'desired' role plays no longer than two to three minutes in length. In Kenya children were divided into 13 groups across three schools, while in Tanzania and South Africa children made four documentaries in total in each country.

To prepare the pupils for this task, they were given instructions and then given a week to prepare and plan their role plays for 'filming' on a prearranged afternoon. Pupils were also energised and excited about doing this task. However, it was not completely plain sailing. In South Africa children struggled with the cameras (we used the video function on normal digital still cameras), and spent much time fooling around, giggling and distracting one another from the task. In Kenya they spent enormous amounts of time role playing detailed stories of AIDS-related tragedies, which were initially difficult to interpret. In Tanzania the quality of videos were far superior because a researcher actually did the filming, whereas in Kenya and South Africa children attempted to do the filming – with variable results. However, the messages in each case were clear, and the data extremely rich and valuable. This activity produced a much better depth and quality of data than, for example, merely interviewing children about current and desired sex and AIDS education. Drawing in additional researchers to assist children with directing (South Africa) and filming (Tanzania) greatly enhanced the activity, although in all three contexts it was a time-consuming task. The data obtained from these mini-video documentaries is discussed in Chapter 6.

Focus group discussions

FGDs were held both with pupils and teachers – on separate occasions. The pupils' FGDs centred on the mini-video documentaries that they had made. They were asked to comment on how realistic their documentaries were in their portrayal of current sex-education classes, whether they felt they had left anything out and, if so, what. These were all successfully conducted, with children becoming quite animated when discussing their documentaries.

The FGDs with teachers covered a number of areas. Teachers were asked to describe the current AIDS education conducted in their schools, to talk about the training they had received in order to teach AIDS education and their struggles in doing so. They were also shown the mini-documentaries made by pupils regarding how they would like AIDS and sex education classes to be taught. Then teachers were asked to comment on how realistic they thought pupils' visions were and how their suggestions might be incorporated into future teaching.

Community dialogues

Community dialogues were convened two to three months after data collection was concluded. This allowed us to transcribe and analyse data, and to decide on core themes across all sites. A PowerPoint presentation was prepared of initial findings, which was then shown to a group of teachers, pupils and community stakeholders in each country. Included in the presentation was a combined and edited video of pupils' desired sex-education mini-documentaries. We made the decision not to show 'current' videos for fear of antagonising teachers through exaggeration. In each country these community dialogues lasted just over two hours, and feedback was either digitally recorded and transcribed or transcribed directly. In South Africa there were 23 participants; in Kenya and Tanzania there were 36 and 35 participants, respectively. Refreshments were served and participants were given a small travel allowance. The school heads were also presented with a digital camera for the school as a token of appreciation for participation in the research study. Most teachers present at these dialogues indicated a willingness to participate in implementing the envisaged toolkit, which we described during our interaction. The data from these dialogues is fully reported in Chapter 7.

Learnings and limitations

In reflecting on the methodological approach employed in this study and on the methods used and challenges encountered, it is possible to offer observations in four areas: working with children on sensitive topics, researching in the midst of poverty, maintaining confidentiality using visual methods and managing data in a three-country study. Each will be considered in turn before recommendations are made on how the study design might have been improved.

Working with children on sensitive topics

When dealing with a culturally and religiously sensitive topic, such as sex education, due care needs to be taken with regard to local sensibilities. This is not to say that researchers ought to avoid broaching topics that are sensitive, but that local informants should always guide discussions. Where it becomes necessary to challenge prevailing norms that are harmful to children this needs to be done in a respectful way (Oluga et al. 2010).

Researching in the midst of poverty

The issue of conducting research in resource-poor communities is seldom reported in literature from the global north. However, more recently, as research grows in impoverished communities increasing numbers of researchers have begun to write about the ethics of working among impoverished communities. Swartz (2009, 2011) draws particular attention to diminishing power gradients, and advocates for research that gives back to communities. In this study especially, the resource-poor context frequently led researchers to become personally, socially and emotionally involved in the lives of participants. For example, in Kenya the researcher made the following entry into her field notes:

> Teachers confided in me about their health. For example, two had breast cancer and I found myself getting both emotionally and financially involved. One teacher wanted me to help get a job for her daughter who had passed her degree with honours but had not yet found a job. I ended up helping her search for job agencies on the internet and advised her to upload her CV. Several teachers asked me if I could help them get visas to the UK…In one school an HIV-positive boy who I had met nine months earlier when doing the rapid ethnography had become so sick that he no longer came to school. I really felt bad for him.

Maintaining confidentiality using visual methods

The use of cameras was an ethical challenge because these pupils were young and mostly from poor communities. Cameras posed several risks to children and their families. Children were at risk of being hurt if someone forcibly stole the camera. Their families feared financial repercussions if cameras were lost, stolen or damaged – although we made it clear that there would be no liability. From the point of view of child protection, these photographs put children at risk of being 'outed' for being an orphan, having an HIV-infected family member, engaging in illicit sex or generally coming to the attention of someone who might harm them. Children were also afraid of people not wanting their photographs taken – although to some extent the training and role plays in how to deal with these situations mitigated these risks. Overall, however, despite almost no adverse incidents, camera use with this age group remains somewhat fraught. Though we have very good photos (and videos), our use of these sources of data is somewhat limited. We can infer from them, but not use them directly or show them to others because of issues of confidentiality. For example, even if the people in the photos gave consent for their pictures to be taken, they can never understand how far their photos may reach through an international audience.

Managing data in a three-country study

This research study produced enormous amounts of data. However, it was an ongoing challenge to ensure that all three contexts followed the agreed research protocol. For example, in Kenya the researcher observed five times more lessons than we had agreed, but then conducted only half as many interviews as had been agreed upon. We had also agreed on using Nvivo (qualitative analysis software) and the same codes for data analysis, but not all researchers were able to use sophisticated software, and demographic data were frequently poorly recorded. It was also difficult to work with data from other contexts because we had allocated one writer to cover different areas within the study rather than one writer per country. Invariably, writers referenced the data they had collected more frequently than that of others, since they had 'been there'. The constant temptation was for the writers to write from the context with which they were most familiar. This resulted in some unevenness in the chapters that follow, which had to be continually revised and reworked.

Overall, however, having three countries with which to compare data has resulted in a rich piece of work with multiple perspectives and a far clearer basis upon which to make recommendations. We have also been able to contrast various contexts that on the surface may appear similar. After all, we were working largely in impoverished primary schools with high pupil-to-teacher ratios and fairly low educational quality. In the chapters that follow it quickly becomes apparent that there are many differences in each context, along with some general principles that apply to all three countries.

Recommendations for future study design

In this chapter we have described our study aims and research questions in some detail, as well as the processes and methods employed to accomplish these aims. On reflection, we would do a few things differently in the future. Our sample might have been smaller and elicited similar data. Asking children to select their peers was a strategy we might have employed across all sites to limit the number of research participants without excluding any by our own selection. We might have worked best if we had a limited amount of time in which to collect data – perhaps not as little as two months, but certainly no more than six. The use of cameras and videos required more training than many of us were able to provide. Many of us as researchers struggled with sophisticated skills that digital photography, video editing and managing data required. Our capacity in these areas needs to be improved.

However, what we have learnt most about is the possibility of consulting pupils by using engaging, interactive and visual methods. When Arnot et al. (2004) and Flutter and Rudduck (2004) revitalised the process of consulting pupils, their methods were largely through interviews. Interactive and visual methods have helped us consult children for whom the conventional interview may have been developmentally inappropriate and may not have elicited the depth of data we have obtained through the visual methods used in this study. Furthermore, we have been surprised by the many ways in which our research design has allowed children, in contexts where talking about sex to adults is a cultural taboo, to speak freely and openly. They have done so with a level of insight for which we were not prepared. The chapters that follow reveal first-hand children's views on how AIDS education programmes in school were, and how they should be, conducted. We have access to teachers' understandings and awareness of young people's contexts and sexual knowledges. We are able to examine the conflicting voices of community stakeholders, who are both aware of the dangers faced by children living in a world with AIDS and afraid of the many cultural, religious and moral restraints to sex education in Africa. The chapters that follow take seriously children's complaints, as captured in one of the South African schools in the study:

> The teachers are careful with us because they think we are still young…They think we are too young to know…They think we are going to be naughty or sometimes experiment what they told us… [but] who wants to experiment with AIDS?

CHAPTER 3

Country context, education policies and AIDS education

As we have described, conducting research in three country contexts presents challenges, but also offers rich data. In this chapter we give a brief description of education in general, and HIV/AIDS education in particular, in each of the countries in which we undertook the research – Kenya, South Africa and Tanzania. These descriptions will help to contextualise and locate the data we report on in the chapters that follow.

Kenya

Kenya experienced high enrolment levels in primary schools immediately after its independence in 1963. Since then there has been a rise in the number of primary schools and enrolment, although between 1989 and 2002 gross enrolment rates fell, with some regions in the north of Kenya having a gross enrolment rate as low as 24 per cent (Bedi et al. 2002). This could be because of a formal cost-sharing system that was introduced in 1988, whereby parents were required to pay for school uniforms, stationery, textbooks, instructional materials and other school equipment. The government's contribution was limited to paying teachers' salaries – a result of the Structural Adjustment Programme imposed on many countries in Africa by the World Bank, intended to speed up economic recovery (Jayahrajah & Branson 1993). In addition, the exponential spread of HIV/AIDS in the country meant that illness and death reduced the ability of a household to pay school fees. Many children stayed at home to become the main caregivers in their homes (Bedi et al. 2002).

Enrolment picked up dramatically with the introduction of free primary education in 2003. This was as a result of, and in response to, the worldwide push for Education For All (KMOEST 2005a), when education came to be seen as a basic right for all Kenyan children and was enshrined in the Children's Act of 2001. There has been a 23.3 per cent increase in enrolment in primary education, from 6 million pupils in 2002 to 7.2 million in 2003 and 8.6 million in 2008 (KMOEST 2009). The government has also now introduced free secondary day tuition for students from poor families (KMOEST 2009). This resulted in a further increase in enrolment in public schools by 18 per cent in 2008 compared to 13.7 per cent in 2007. Predictably, the system was not ready for such an influx of children, and problems of over-crowding, and a lack of sufficient infrastructure, teachers and teaching resources were experienced. International donor and development organisations have contributed funds towards bridging the immediate funding shortfalls, especially those related to teaching and learning materials. These organisations include UNESCO, UNICEF, the Swedish International Development Agency, the Department for International Development, the World Bank, the Canadian International Development Agency, the World Food Program, the Japan International Cooperation Agency, and the Deutsche Gesellschaft für Technische Zusammenarbeit. Most of these donors are now part of the Kenya Education Sector Support

Programme (KESSP) 2005–2010, which comprises 23 investment programmes. KESSP operationalises the budget for prioritised programmes, which, when accomplished, will ensure that agreed goals and objectives are attained (Eastern Africa Network of HIV/AIDS & Education in Eastern Africa 2010). The Kenyan government has also put in place two policies, the Education Sector Support Program 2005–2015 and the Education Sector Strategic Plan 2003–2007 which spell out plans for improving access, transition and completion rates (KMOEST 2005b). They also address issues such as school-based teacher development, curriculum reform and investment in capacity building (KMOEST 2005b).

However, there are still between 2.1 and 2.6 million children of school-going age who are out of school, the majority of whom are child workers (Manda et al. 2003; United Nations Integrated Regional Information Networks 2006). Although it is considered a success to enrol more children in schools, it has been a challenge for teachers to control large classes, usually resulting in lecture-type teaching and little room for interactive pedagogy. At the beginning of the school year in 2003, hundreds of thousands of children showed up at primary schools, many of them desperately poor, with no clothes or shoes, and nothing to write with or on. Most of them had never been to school. Class sizes swelled from 40 to between 70 and 100. Children were learning in shifts, with some attending in the morning and some in the afternoon (Mathooko 2009). The situation seems to have stabilised since then with the help of donor funding and the implementation of strategic plans.

Education at different levels

Most children start primary education at the age of six. Pre-school education in support of early child-hood development (ECD) is not compulsory and depends largely on the child's family. In Kenya, the government does not hire ECD teachers and does not run ECD schools. They are mostly private or run by churches and the community. However, the government said it will aim to recruit ECD teachers and support the provision of teaching and learning materials by 2010 – but this has yet to happen. There are eight years of primary education (standards 1 to 8), four years of secondary education (forms 1 to 4), and four years of university education; hence the term '8-4-4' for the Kenyan education system. There are 12 subjects in the primary education curriculum: mathematics, English, Kiswahili, science, social studies, Christian religious education, Hindu religious education, Islamic religious education, creative arts, physical education, mother tongue, and life skills education. Mother Tongue is taught from standard 1 to 3; all the other subjects are taught from standard 1 to 8. Kenyans speak several languages, including the official languages (English and Kiswahili) and indigenous languages, including Kikuyu (spoken by 22 per cent); Luhya (14 per cent); Luo (13 per cent); Kalenjin (12 per cent); Kamba (11 per cent); Kisii (6 per cent); Meru (6 per cent); other African languages (15 per cent); and non-African languages (Asian, European and Arab – 1 per cent) (Central Intelligence Agency 2010). The Kenya National Examinations Council examines all the subjects taught at the end of standard 8, except for creative arts, physical education, mother tongue and life skills. Religious education is elective, with pupils learning their nominated religion. Religious affiliation in Kenya is as follows: Protestant (45 per cent); Roman Catholic (33 per cent); Muslim (10 per cent); indigenous beliefs (10 per cent); and other (2 per cent) (Central Intelligence Agency 2010). At the end of each phase, the pupil sits for a national exam to qualify for transition to the next phase. For example, at the end of standard 8 they sit for the Kenya Certificate for Primary Education and at the end of secondary school (form 4), they sit for the Kenya Certificate for Secondary Education. Table 3.1 summarises numbers of educational institutions and enrolments as of 2008. In 2008, KMOEST (2009) reported that only 75.3 per cent of girls had completed the full cycle of primary education at standard 8, compared to 85.1 per cent of boys. The public primary schools had the most teachers (170 059), compared to public secondary schools (43 016) and early childhood development schools (78 230). The teacher:pupil ratio was 22.2:1 for early childhood development schools; 44.6:1 for primary schools; and 32:1 for secondary schools (KMOEST 2009).

TABLE 3.1 *Number of educational institutions and enrolments in Kenya (as of 2008)*

Type of institution	Number	Enrolment
Early childhood development schools	37 954	1.72 million
Primary schools	26 206 (of these, 1 574 have special-needs education institutions)	8.56 million (boys 51 per cent, girls 49 per cent)
Secondary schools	6 566	1.38 million (boys 54 per cent, girls 46 per cent)
Primary teacher-training colleges	36	222 000 (male 51 per cent, female 49 per cent)
Universities	28	122 800 (male 60 per cent, female 40 per cent)

Source: Data from KMOEST (2009)

The HIV/AIDS pandemic

The first reported case of HIV in Kenya was in 1984 (Muraah & Kiarie 2001; Nyaga et al. 2004). The nickname then for the virus was 'slim' because it was associated with weight loss of those infected (Muraah & Kiarie 2001; Nyaga et al. 2004). At first, the Kenyan government took a defensive stand against any suggestions of HIV/AIDS spreading in Kenya, but the escalating pandemic made it impossible for the government to continue in its denial, and in 1985 the government set up the National AIDS Council within the Ministry of Health. In 1990 out of a consortium of non-governmental organisations (NGOs), the Kenya AIDS NGOs Consortium (KANCO) became the main organisation for spearheading efforts for cooperation between the state and civil society, mostly through its advocacy and policy initiatives (KANCO 2008). AIDS was recognised as a 'national disaster' by the government in 1999 (Ahlberg & Pertet 2006: 8). This use of the language of security, which accorded HIV/AIDS the serious attention it deserved, was an acknowledgement that the epidemic was adversely affecting every aspect of Kenyan society and that it would require a more direct response in terms of policies and financial resources (Wambuii 2006: 62). The president set up the National AIDS Control Council, which was mandated to coordinate efforts in the prevention and control of HIV/AIDS in Kenya.

The principal mode of HIV/AIDS transmission in Kenya (i.e. 75 per cent) is heterosexual contact (Kenya Demographic and Health Survey 2003). HIV prevalence in Kenya has gradually decreased from 15 per cent in 2001 to 6.1 per cent in 2006 owing to behaviour change, such as 15- to 24-year-olds having fewer non-regular sex partners, and women reporting an increased use of condoms (Kenya Demographic and Health Survey 2003). More recently, this prevalence rate has increased to 7.8 per cent (adults aged 15–64). A reason offered for this rise is the increased use of antiretroviral drugs (ARVs), resulting in a fall in AIDS-related deaths of 29 per cent since 2002 (UNAIDS/WHO 2009). Furthermore, those taking ARVs were thought to be having an increased number of sexual partners after regaining their health (Gathura & Okwemba 2008).[2] The most recently available UNAIDS data report a falling prevalence rate of 6.3 per cent for adults aged 15 to 49 (UNAIDS/WHO 2010), which indicates that the rate of new infections in fact remains somewhat static. However, unprotected sex among youth remains a concern in Kenya. It is reported that a typical young person in Kenya becomes sexually active between the ages of 15 and 19, and fewer than 25 per cent of them will use a condom the first time they have sex (National

2   Gathura G & Okwemba A, Kenya losing the fight against HIV after all, experts warn, *The Daily Nation*, 29 July 2008, http://www.nation.co.ke/News/-/1056/444870/-/view/printVersion/-/y800kfz/-/index.html.

AIDS/STI Control Programme 2006, as cited in UNAIDS/WHO 2009). The rate of infection is especially disproportionate for girls and young women. Women between 15 and 19 are three times more likely to be infected than their male counterparts, and 20- to 24-year-old women are 5.5 times more likely to be living with HIV than men in their age cohort (National AIDS/STI Control Programme 2006, as cited in UNAIDS/WHO 2009). This may be the result of younger women taking older sexual partners.

HIV/AIDS education

In 1999 when HIV/AIDS was declared a national disaster, HIV/AIDS education was made a stand-alone subject in the national curriculum. Consequently, the Kenya Institute of Education developed a series of handbooks for teachers and students, e.g. *AIDS education facilitators' handbook* ; *AIDS education syllabus for schools and colleges* ; *Bloom or doom: Your choice* ; *Let us talk about AIDS: A book for Class 1, 2 and 3* ; *Let us talk about AIDS: A book for Class 4 and 5* ; and *Let us talk about AIDS: A book for Class 6, 7 and 8* (Eastern Africa Network of HIV/AIDS & Education in Eastern Africa 2010). These books aimed to equip students with the necessary knowledge, attitudes and skills to avoid being infected with HIV and other sexually transmitted infections. The aim was to develop students as responsible citizens who could make rational decisions for themselves (Eastern Africa Network of HIV/AIDS & Education in Eastern Africa 2010). However, this initiative failed and after one year, HIV/AIDS education was removed from the timetable, mainly because teachers were not prepared to teach about sex – considered a sensitive topic. A new curriculum was designed in 2002, infusing HIV/AIDS information in other 'carrier' subjects, and schools are now also required to have one HIV/AIDS lesson per week.

HIV/AIDS policy

Several HIV/AIDS policies have been designed in various sectors. Sessional Paper No. 4 (KMOEST 1997) provided a policy framework to guide all partners in Kenya's response to the challenges of HIV/AIDS. For example, some teacher training colleges, such as Kagumo Teacher's College and Highridge Teacher's College, have their own policies which articulate a vision of the colleges' commitment to integrating HIV/AIDS into its curriculum – teaching, research, co-curricular activities and community services; the acknowledgement of the rights and responsibilities of the infected and the affected in the colleges; and an openness to dialogue and reviews. The government has also designed the Kenyan National HIV/AIDS Strategic Plan 2005/06–2009/10 (KNACC 2005), which has an overall theme of social change to reduce HIV/AIDS and poverty. It provides the framework and context within which strategies, plans and budgets should be formulated, monitored and coordinated. The Education Sector Policy on HIV and AIDS (KMOEST 2004) aims to facilitate broader understanding and strengthen partnerships between education service providers in the fight against the pandemic. The HIV and AIDS workplace policy for the public sector aims to provide guidance on the management of employees who are infected and affected by HIV and AIDS and to prevent further infections. It outlines employees' responsibilities, rights and expected behaviour (Eastern Africa Network of HIV/AIDS & Education in Eastern Africa 2010). Other supportive policies include a policy on condom use, national guidelines on voluntary counselling and testing, guidelines on national home-based care programmes and services, and guidelines on blood safety, ARV treatment and on preventing mother-to-child transmission.

South Africa

Under the Apartheid government, education in South Africa was differentiated along racial lines. White children received the best education in terms of academic content, physical facilities and ratio of teachers to students; black children received the worst. In between was education for coloured and Indian children. The infamous Bantu Education Act (No. 48 of 1953) wrote into law the mandate of 'education for servitude' – educating black children only for a future as labourers or 'servants' in a white-dominated country. The then minister of education, Hendrik Verwoerd held that '[t]here is no place for [the black African] in the European community above the level of certain forms of labour. It is of no avail for him to receive a training which has as its aim absorption in the European community.'[3]

At the height of Apartheid in 1975, social spending (including spending on education) on black South Africans was less than 12 per cent of that spent on white youth (Terreblanche 2002: 389). The consequence of Apartheid education is described by David Everatt (1994: 3):

> The Apartheid education system was premised on under-educating black South Africans, and on ejecting them from the education system very early. Outside that system, life for young black South Africans was marked by structural violence, including denial of decent employment, housing and family life. The lived experience which flowed from this structural violence has led to substance abuse, political violence, rape, teenage pregnancies and the other well-known consequences of this type of situation.

After the first democratic elections of 1994, transforming the education system in South Africa became a priority. The National Department of Basic Education is responsible for primary- and high-school education across the country and provides a national framework for school policy. Provincial departments are responsible for implementing this policy, and at local school level, elected school governing bodies assist in local schools (Government Communication and Information Services 2009). Post-1994 school infrastructure[4] was prioritised, and there was a thorough revision of curriculum content and pedagogy. Money spent on education in South Africa amounts to 17.8 per cent of total government expenditure (R92.1 billion in 2006). However, of this amount, a large proportion is spent on school nutrition programmes, and does not go into traditional features associated with ensuring children obtain a high-quality education.

There have also been a number of new national curriculum frameworks and approaches over the 17 years of South Africa's democracy. However, education quality in South Africa remains poor, especially for the majority who still attend township schools, and more especially in rural areas and poorer provinces.[5] The result is that, for example, South African children score lowest on international numeracy and literacy standards, frequently lower than poorer African neighbouring countries.

So while children are now free to attend any school, variables such as distances between township homes and good suburban schools, language policies in schools and school fees frequently militate against poor children receiving a decent-quality education. There are currently 25 875 schools in South Africa, of which 1 124 (4.3 per cent) are independent schools (DoE 2009: 6). Therefore, the vast majority of South African children attend state-funded schools. These schools are ranked into five quintiles according to

---

3   South Africa History Online (2008) *The youth struggle – Education in South Africa*, http://www.sahistory.org.za/pages/governance-projects/june16/bantu-edu.htm.
4   Seventy-one per cent of all primary schools have 'reliable water'; 69 per cent have 'decent sanitation'; and 76 per cent have access to 'reliable electricity' (South Africa Government Communication and Information Services 2009: 170).
5   The greatest educational challenges lie in the poorer, rural provinces, like the Eastern Cape and KwaZulu-Natal. Schools are generally better resourced in the more affluent provinces, such as Gauteng and the Western Cape.

the level of poverty experienced in the communities in which they are located. Quintile 1 schools are the poorest; schools in quintile 5 are the least poor. In our study School A was ranked quintile 3 and School B was (somewhat optimistically) ranked quintile 5. Schools in quintiles 1 to 3 are particularly targeted with the National School Nutrition Programme, in which learners receive a meal a day while at school. As far as government expenditure is concerned, there are intentional polices that require provinces to spend more money on poorer schools and less on wealthier schools. So, for example, the poorest 20 per cent of learners receive 35 per cent of non-personnel resources, while the richest 20 per cent receive 5 per cent (Government Communication and Information Services 2009: 169).

Language

South Africa has 11 official languages, all of which are given equal status, but vary in terms of the extent to which they are used in each of the nine provinces. Language policy in South African schools since 1994 provides that education at the primary level (Grades R–7) is conducted in the child's home language, while in secondary school education is provided in either English or Afrikaans. Students who write the national school-leaving examinations are entitled to a 5 per cent allowance if they are African first-language candidates who write the examinations in their second language (i.e. English or Afrikaans). These students, however, continue to achieve at a rate far below their first-language counterparts (Umalusi 2004).

Compulsory schooling, enrolment and fees

There are two official school-leaving points, the first at the end of Grade 9 (National Qualifications Framework (NQF) Level 1) and the second at Grade 12, or matric (NQF Level 4). According to the National Education Policy Act (No. 27 of 1996), school is compulsory for all children from 7 to 15 (usually Grades 1–9). Grade R is not compulsory and neither are Grades 10–12. According to United Nations data for the period 2003–2008 (UNICEF 2010), at the primary level South Africa has gross[6] universal enrolment (105 per cent for boys and 101 per cent for girls). The net[7] enrolment rate is lower, at 86 per cent. Furthermore, 77 per cent of children who enrol for primary education in Grade 1 reach Grade 5. The secondary-school enrolment rate is 93 per cent (gross), 70 per cent (net) for males, and 99 per cent (gross), 75 per cent (net) for females. Only 50 per cent of students who enrol for Grade 1 exit Grade 12 (DoE 2009). There is overall gender parity with regard to school enrolment at both primary and secondary levels (DoE 2009: 8).

With regard to school retention, the matric pass rate, which was as low as 40 per cent in the late 1990s, continues to improve each year, reaching 68.3 per cent in 2005. Disparity remains among 'race groups' with regard to school completion and pass rates. Whereas 65 per cent of white people over 20 years old and 40 per cent of Indians have a high-school or higher qualification, this figure is only 14 per cent among black people and 17 per cent among the coloured population (Statistics South Africa 2001).

School fees, set by the school governing body, are charged at all schools. However, there are a number of schools designated by the minister of education as being no-fee schools. This is announced from time to time. Theoretically, schools are not permitted to exclude children on the basis of not being able to pay school fees. In 2010, 64 per cent of all government-funded schools were so designated (Government Communication and Information Services 2009: 170). Neither are they permitted to be excluded from any school on the basis of race or religion. Some schools do, however, have entrance

6   Gross school enrolment rate defines the number of children enrolled in a level (primary or secondary), regardless of age, divided by the population of the age group that officially corresponds to the same level.
7   Net primary school enrolment rate is the number of children enrolled in primary school that belong to the age group that officially corresponds to primary schooling, divided by the total population of the same age group.

exams in which, for example, language ability is tested. Well-resourced schools frequently depend on substantial schools fees being paid by parents, which fund additional teachers in order to reduce teacher:student ratios, attract high-quality teachers and pay for additional coaching and instruction for extramural activities. These schools are accused of covertly excluding students because of their inability to pay top-up fees.

Religions

According to the 2001 census (Statistics South Africa 2001), the overwhelming majority of South Africans (79.8 per cent) are Christian. The independent African Zion Christian churches predominate – the faith of 15.3 per cent of the total population and 19.2 per cent of all Christians. Roughly 15 per cent of the population have no religion, and 1.4 per cent are undetermined about their faith. Islam is the religion of 1.5 per cent of South Africans; Hinduism that of 1.2 per cent; African traditional belief 0.3 per cent; Judaism 0.2 per cent; and other beliefs 0.6 per cent.

TABLE 3.2 *Religions in South Africa*

Religion	Number	%
Christianity	35 766 180	79.8
Islam	672 297	1.5
Hinduism	537 837	1.2
Judaism	89 640	0.2
African traditional belief	134 459	0.3
Other beliefs	268 919	0.6
No religion	6 722 966	15
Undetermined	627 477	1.4
Total	44 819 774	100

Source: Statistics South Africa (2001)

In line with the Constitution of the Republic of South Africa, the National Education Policy Act states: 'Every learner and educator shall have the right to freedom of conscience, religion, thought, belief, opinion, speech and expression and the education process shall promote a culture of tolerance.' Religious observances at public schools have been ensured through the South African Schools Act (No. 84 of 1996). The Act offers guarantees for conducting religious observances at public schools provided that such practices are done fairly and attendance at them by pupils and staff is free and optional. Religious education is taught at both primary and secondary levels, and focuses on mean- ing in life, the affirmation of the learner's religious identity and an informed respect for the religious identity of others. It aims to 'recognise diversity...[and] foster tolerance, respect and understanding' (Government Communication and Information Services 2009: 171).

HIV/AIDS figures

The latest HIV/AIDS statistics show that in 2009 the prevalence for the 15–49 age group was 17.8 per cent in South Africa (UNAIDS/WHO 2010). In 2008 the national prevalence of HIV among children under 18 was 2.9 per cent, with similar prevalence for boys and girls (Shisana et al. 2010). Prevalence was highest among adolescents 15–18 years of age at 4.5 per cent and 0–4-year-olds, at 3.3 per cent. It was 2.5 per cent for those 5–11 years of age and 1.1 per cent for teenagers 12–14 years of age. For children under 14, infection is largely a 'result of vertical transmission (from mother to child), where the prevalence is high among children 0–4 years of age, and HIV prevalence declines due to HIV/AIDS-related mortality among those 5–11 and 12–14 years of age' (UNAIDS/WHO 2010: 31). The prevalence estimate for these children was lowest in the rural formal areas (1.9 per cent) and highest in the urban informal areas (4.5 per cent).

National HIV/AIDS policy as it relates to education

Sexuality and life skills education has become the educational response to the HIV pandemic and is included in both primary and secondary education as a component of life orientation. The two key policies outlining the educational response to the AIDS pandemic are contained in the National Policy on HIV and AIDS for Learners and Educators in Public Schools and Students and Educators in Further Education and Training Institutions (DoE 1999), and the HIV and AIDS Emergency Guidelines for Educators (DoE 2000a). The Department of Health's National Strategic Plan for HIV and AIDS and Sexually Transmitted Infections (STIs) (Department of Health 2007) includes a special focus on prevention efforts targeting youth aged 15 to 24. These plans include using schools as centres of care and support, as well as monitoring and evaluating school-based interventions.

In terms of curricula, HIV/AIDS and sexuality are key content areas in life orientation, a programme that was introduced as a learning area in South African schools in the late 1990s (DoE 2002c; Rooth, 2005). Life orientation comprises several components: guidance, life-skills education, health promotion, physical development and movement, environmental education, citizenship and human rights education, and religious education. Schools and teachers are allowed autonomy in terms of what they teach and what they omit.

In 2001 the Department of Education (DoE 2002b) convened a conference to discuss the values that should underpin sexuality education in schools. In the resulting report, *Protecting the right to innocence: The importance of sexuality education*, it was concluded that these values needed to be 'personal responsibility, respect for self and others, a regard for human rights and gender equity' (DoE 2002b: 23). The report also provided the framework in which sexuality education was to be taught – not as a stand-alone subject, but as part of the broader life-skills focus. Teacher training was emphasised, as was the need to 'listen to children' in matters regarding sexuality.

Subsequently, according to the National Curriculum Statement for Grades R–9 (South DoE 2002c), the curriculum contains strategies for 'dealing with HIV/AIDS and nurturing a culture of sexual and social responsibility' (DoE 2002c: 8). In particular, it aims to ensure that learners are 'able to make informed decisions regarding personal, community and environmental health' (DoE 2002c: 26). The Life Orientation Curriculum Statement (DoE 2002a) for primary-aged learners places emphasis during the foundation phase (Grades 0–3) on being aware of the existence of HIV as a disease and being able to 'avoid sexual abuse and report it' (DoE 2002a: 12). At the intermediate level (Grades 4–6), sex and HIV/AIDS education is focused on combating gender stereotypes and sexism, as well as understanding the 'causes of communicable diseases (including HIV/AIDS) and available cures', and being able to evaluate 'prevention strategies, in relation to community norms and personal values' (DoE 2002a: 29). In the senior phase (Grade 7 onwards) learners ought to be able to 'describe strategies for living with diseases, including HIV/AIDS' and discuss 'the personal feelings, community norms, values and social pressures associated with sexuality' (DoE 2002a: 40). The emphasis on community norms is frequently repeated, but little other guidance is provided in the curriculum statements. Such guidance may be available elsewhere, but is not part of the formal curriculum policy documents available from the South African Department of Basic Education.

In a study that considered the way in which teachers interacted with HIV-related policies (Simbayi et al., 2005) it was found that educators were aware of the policies that governed education and management of HIV/AIDS, but felt that policies failed to adequately address stigma, and were inadequately operationalised within the school environment. In addition, about half of the educators surveyed reported having taught learners about HIV/AIDS. Teachers who taught about AIDS were mainly senior, white and coloured, and had read the Department's policies. In addition, although most teachers were willing to teach learners about human sexuality and safe-sex practices, white educators were not so keen to teach learners about the use of condoms.

Teacher preparation policies and processes

In 1994, the democratic government of South Africa inherited a highly fragmented and unresponsive education system. One of the first steps taken by government was to rationalise the number of institutions providing in-service and pre-service teacher education following a national audit in 1995. These institutions included universities, technikons, colleges of education, private colleges, and NGOs. The audit also concluded that the quality of teacher education was generally poor, inefficient and not cost-effective. Subsequently, and in alignment with international trends, colleges of education were incorporated into existing universities and technikons, and the number of institutions providing teacher education dropped from 120 to 50 in 1994, and to 20 by 2005.

Policy on curricula for teacher education has also shifted in focus from content to competence (DoE 2000b). In terms of this policy, teacher education curricula must ensure that theory and practice are integrated. Initial training of teachers is now an integrated 480-credit degree, the BEd. Parallel to this qualification, but at a lower level and catering for older, underqualified teachers, is the National Professional Diploma in Education. Little funding is available, however, for in-service training, and underqualified teachers remain in the system. Also affected by the lack of funding is the limited amount of school-based teaching experience and on-site assessment of practical teaching competence for new teachers.

The implications of this state of affairs for HIV and sexuality education are obvious. Teachers struggle to cope with innovation, and also face cultural hurdles regarding community standards and taboos. As a result, teachers teach technical knowledge and not sexuality education, which embraces both a discourse of 'desire and disease' (Francis 2010). In addition, their pedagogical skills are poorly developed and they receive minimal training to tackle youth needs concerning the complexities of the HIV pandemic. Despite the many places in which teacher education is highlighted as a means of improving education quality in general, and the effective teaching of sexuality education in particular, teacher education with regard to sex and HIV/AIDS education seems to be promoted through workshops and day-long conferences. Teachers also frequently follow perceived community norms and values, and omit important parts of the stated curricular goals.

Tanzania

The United Republic of Tanzania consists of mainland Tanzania and the islands of Zanzibar and Pemba. Tanzania's annual population growth is 3 per cent. In 2004, the population was estimated to be 37.6 million (World Bank 2006), with just under half (43 per cent) of the population estimated to be aged 14 or younger in 2005 (UNSTATS 2005). There are some 120 ethnic groups in Tanzania and their religious affiliation can be broken down into three broad groups: Christian, Muslim and traditionalist.

TABLE 3.3 *Proportions of religious adherents in Tanzania, by source*

Religion	Pew Forum 2009 (%)	Census 1967 (%)	Demographic Health Survey 2004 (%)	Afrobaro-meter 2008 (%)
Christian	60	34	57	63
Muslim	36	31	30	29
Other/none	4	35	13	8

Source: Pew Forum on Religion & Public Life (2010) *Islam and Christianity in sub-Saharan Africa.* Appendix B: Religious demography of sub-Saharan Africa. http://pewforum.org/religious-demography-islam-and-christianity-in-sub-saharan-africa.aspx

Detailed census data about religious adherence has been unavailable since this item was removed from the government census in 1967. However, in a recent survey conducted by the Pew Forum[8] it was estimated that 60 per cent of the population are Christian, 36 per cent Muslim and 4 per cent other/none. Commentators usually attribute the category of other/none to those who are predominantly traditionalists and follow African traditional religions. Table 3.3 provides a breakdown by source and includes data from the last census that included religious affiliation, which described the population as evenly split between Christian, Muslim and other/none (or traditionalists).

Tanzania has two official languages, English and Kiswahili; Kiswahili is the most widely used of the two. However, there are more than 120 tribal languages spoken in Tanzania, which fall into three major language categories: Bantu, Nile Hermitic and Khoisan. The language of instruction in primary school is Kiswahili; English is taught as a foreign language. In secondary and tertiary education, however, the medium of instruction is English. Recently there have been calls to use English as the main medium of instruction in primary schools. Most of the secondary teachers report switching between English and Kiswahili in the classroom owing to limited confidence in English (Tanzania Ministry of Education and Culture 2000).

Basic education

Basic education in Tanzania is made up of seven years of primary schooling (Standards 1–7), which is universal and compulsory. The average age of pupils on entry into Standard 1 is seven. The net enrolment rate in 2007/08 was 97.2 per cent and the gender parity index 0.99 (m = 97.5; f = 97.0). The dropout rate fluctuated between 3.2 per cent in 2003 and 3.7 per cent in 2008 (Tanzania Ministry of Educational and Vocational Training 2008). Enrolment has increased significantly owing to the introduction of the Primary Education Development Plan in 2001 and the cessation of primary-school fees (TESDP 2009). In 2002 alone, Standard 1 enrolment increased by 43.1 per cent. Between 2000 and 2002, around 1.7 million additional children enrolled in primary schools (Mushi et al. 2003). However, many schools have had to adopt double-shift teaching to cope with the increased enrolment. This has led to a fall in teaching hours from 6 to 3.5 per day. The existing primary-school teacher to pupil ratio was 1:54 in 2008, whereas the required national ratio is 1:45 (Tanzania Ministry of Educational and Vocational Training 2008). The achievement and quality of education in Tanzania is officially measured by a final national examination. The pass rate for the Primary School Leaving Examination in 2008 was 52.7 per cent (Tanzania Ministry of Educational and Vocational Training 2008). Critics have argued that this pass rate – higher than in the past – is due to an increased weighting of marks for Kiswahili, with a concomitant decrease in the weighting of mathematics and English for the examination (Davidson 2005).

8   Pew Forum on Religion & Public Life (2010) *Islam and Christianity in sub-Saharan Africa.* Appendix B: Religious demography of sub-Saharan Africa, http://pewforum.org/religious-demography-islam-and-christianity-in-sub-saharan-africa.aspx.

Secondary education

The secondary school has two cycles. The first cycle, Ordinary Level (or lower secondary), lasts for four years and spans Forms I to IV. The second cycle is Forms V and VI, and is termed Advanced Level (or upper secondary). The median commencement age is 15 for lower secondary (Form 1) and 19 for upper secondary (Form V). The annual fee for day secondary school per student is Tsh20 000 ($15.00) and for boarding school Tsh75 000 ($56.00). This excludes the costs of uniforms, textbooks, stationery (pens and writing books) and transport to school. The secondary-school system has grown considerably over the past five years; much of this growth can be accounted for by community-built government day schools. The number of secondary schools that are registered has increased from 3 485 in 2007 to 3 793 in 2008 (TESDP 2009). The total number of Forms I to VI students increased from 1 020 510 (477 314 female; 543 196 male) in 2007 to 1 222 403 (543 279 female; 679 124 male) in 2008. This is an increase of 19.3 per cent. Therefore, secondary education gross enrolment (Forms I to VI) increased from 22.1 per cent in 2007 to 26.1 per cent in 2008 (TESDP 2009). This is attributed to the increased number of secondary schools constructed by communities.

Teacher education

A Certificate of Teaching is required to teach in a primary school, and the minimum admission requirement for teacher training is a division III qualification at the O-level examination. There are four divisions, I to IV, with I the highest and IV the lowest before a fail. The language of instruction for the certificate of teaching is Kiswahili. For teaching secondary level, a diploma is required and a degree qualification is needed for upper-secondary teaching. However, the quality of secondary-school teachers is low, as Osaki and Njabili (reported in Wedgwood 2005: 34) comment:

> At diploma level most trainees enter with a mixture of Ds and Es, and many with only 2 E grades. In practice this means that many trainees lack understanding of the fundamental concepts that they are expected to teach. Even with such a low entry point, teacher training colleges cannot fill all their places.

It is well known that most secondary schools in Tanzania are understaffed and the understaffing is worse in community-built secondary schools.

HIV/AIDS: Policy and status in Tanzania

Tanzania is among the sub-Saharan African countries widely affected by HIV/AIDS. Recent statistics put HIV prevalence for adults aged between 15 and 49 at 5.6 per cent (compared to 7.1 in 2001) (UNAIDS/WHO 2010). Of these, 70.5 per cent were in the age group 25–49, and 15 per cent were aged 15-24 (Tanzania Prime Minister's Office 2001). Therefore, AIDS is one of the leading causes of death in young adults in Tanzania.

In dealing with the AIDS problem, the Tanzanian government established the Tanzania Commission on AIDS to provide leadership and coordinate responses from a wide range of groups. As education is seen as a social determinant of health, Tanzania's Ministry of Education decided to develop education sector policies and guidelines in 2004, which set principles and goals for prevention, treatment, care and support. The basic principle of the policy is the mainstreaming of HIV-related prevention education in all educational sectors. The strength of the policy is that HIV-prevention education is incorporated into the official school curriculum from primary to secondary school. However, the main threat, acknowledged by the Ministry of Education, is that the lack of training for teachers could lead to inadequate teaching of sexuality and HIV/AIDS in the curriculum (Tanzania Ministry of Education and Culture 2004).

CHAPTER 4

A rapid ethnography of contexts and AIDS education

Research in developing countries has emphasised the importance of the school in terms of its influence on pupil learning, suggesting that it has more effect than the home and other external factors, which are the dominant influences in developed countries (Ackers & Hardman 2001; Hardman et al. 2008; Scheerens 2000; Verspoor 2003). Within the school, the classroom pedagogy and school climate are the crucial elements that shape learning. Hardman et al. (2008) have shown that teachers are often under-prepared in pedagogical matters during their initial teacher education and consequently lack confidence. Therefore, these authors argue that it is important to study pedagogy at the school and classroom level. These elements, together with our emphasis on the interaction between everyday and school knowledge (Bernstein 1990a, 1999) make it essential to gain a sense of the school as a context for this research.

Teachers and students are situated in communities that influence their understandings, their confidence to explore certain topics and the school's practices. The contextual sketch provided in this chapter might help us to understand further the barriers to teachers' use of everyday knowledge in their practice. Our aim was to understand and document the important interaction between the knowledges that young people bring to the classroom and the formal messages disseminated by teachers and policy-makers. To realise this aim we needed to pay attention to the discourses in the school and the classroom where HIV/AIDS education was taking place. Our hope was that by engaging as fully as possible with the underlying issues, difficulties and dilemmas faced by teachers as agents of sexual knowledge, and about schools as spaces of sexual knowledge we might be able to offer new strategies for pedagogical practice.

Rapid ethnography

In the previous chapter, we provided some of the statistics about children's macro-contexts. In this chapter, we move to the level of what we were able to observe first-hand about homes, schooling, poverty and social environments, before proceeding to what we were told. Although all three of these elements are critical to achieve an understanding of the sociocultural context, here we employed a technique known as rapid ethnography (described in Chapter 2) to understand children's immediate contexts. Rapid ethnographies were conducted in the three countries and in each of the eight schools we identified as research sites: Mombasa, Kenya (three schools); Cape Town, South Africa (two schools); and Dar es Salaam, Tanzania (three schools). Rapid ethnography involved the researchers spending three to five days per school and making observations of the community setting or locality; the school as a physical space; classroom teaching, especially HIV-related education; and undertaking informal interviews as well as getting to know the teachers, pupils and related community members associated with the schools. Data presented here are drawn from all eight schools. There are similarities among the schools, but also some notable differences. This discussion focuses on two main aspects: first, the characteristics of the community in which the school is located and, second, the school as a context for HIV/AIDS education.

Homes, communities and schools

The physical environments in which the children lived shared a common feature of being economically disadvantaged. For the most, the poverty markers include the types of houses and homes in which young people lived; levels of unemployment, crime and substance abuse in the communities; the availability of recreational spaces; cultural and religious practices; school resources; attendance levels; feeding schemes; and the impact of HIV/AIDS on communities. Although specific contexts varied considerably between countries and even between the sites in each country, these elements were common to all the sites. Each will be considered in turn.

Houses and homes

With regard to housing, in Cape Town, pupils attending School A lived predominantly in shacks constructed of corrugated iron sheets, cardboard and wood in an informal settlement with shared toilets and taps. The school, however, was well resourced and in a more developed part of the black township with tarred roads, small brick houses and a functioning rubbish-collection system. A current phenomenon in South African township communities is that those who are able to afford better-quality schooling send their children to schools in nearby suburbs (formerly white areas), and their places in local schools are taken by children from other nearby informal settlements. Many inhabitants of informal settlements are newly arrived from rural areas of South Africa or from neighbouring counties, and include those who are chronically unemployed. Pupils from School B in Cape Town lived across the highway in a particularly impoverished part of a historically coloured community. Here houses were slightly larger than those surrounding School A in the township and were predominantly semi-detached four-roomed council houses that had indoor taps and flush toilets.

In the two urban sites in Mombasa (Schools B and C), most children lived in slums in a single-roomed, mud-walled house with no sanitation facilities. In both these communities there were open sewers and large rubbish dumps in the streets, evidence of the lack of a waste-collection system. The rural Kenyan site (School A) was similarly impoverished, although there was more space around the shacks. The site was about half a kilometre from a very large rubbish dump, where children could be seen hanging from lorries delivering rubbish and where people lived in houses made from the rubbish (see Photo 1).

In Tanzania the localities were a mixture of slums and lower- and middle-class homes. Most of the children came from what are commonly recognised as lower-class homes, and in most cases occupied just a room or two in a shared rented house. Seventy per cent of the children in Tanzania in this study lived in rented rooms.

As a result of living in close proximity to others due to poverty and small living spaces, children were frequently exposed to sexual activity at an early age. Children of both sexes often shared rooms or slept with parents. In most cases, children lived in single-parent homes, seldom with both parents. Some young single parents lived with their children in their family's home. Many children from divorced or separated families, those who were orphaned or born to single parents, lived with grandparents, frequently in crowded surroundings. From a purely structural perspective, those who lived in environments with outside and shared toilets were inevitably exposed to the dangers of sexual assault and of other sexual acts.

Levels of crime, unemployment and substance use

Crime was a commonly identified problem in Cape Town in both black and coloured communities. A researcher (near School B in the coloured area) was advised by a taxi driver to hide her mobile phone in her bra and to walk on the main road as if familiar with the area. Later when another researcher visited School A, this time a male, he was advised to take a taxi rather than a train in order to avoid the lengthy walk to the school and lessen the probability of being robbed. In South Africa, it was reported that much crime was committed by young people, some of whom were school dropouts and/or unemployed. Crime involved housebreaking, street muggings, drug trafficking and fighting between two rival gangs, known as 'Stupas' and 'Money Makers', in the area near School B, and more than five gangs near School A. It was reported that gang members, who stand on street corners plying their trade, frequently end up in violent fights over territory.

The researchers in Tanzania did not report any overt crime in their communities, but instead reported a strong sense of neighbourliness (*Ujamaa*) among community members. This sense of neighbourliness was also reported in Mombasa, although residents in the slums complained of theft, prostitution and people drinking the locally brewed *mnazi* (coconut brew). Throughout Kenya, Mombasa is known as a relatively safe place. The researcher experienced dropping her phone twice in two different places only to go back and find that someone had kept it safe for her.

In all three countries it was expressed that substance abuse (both drugs and alcohol) and 'prostitution' (as participants termed sex work) were growing problems. School A in Tanzania was situated in an area renowned for nightly commercial sex activity, and was close to a number of illegal brothels. However, it was predominantly in Cape Town that crime and substance abuse were both visible to the researcher and apparent to participants. Children spoke regularly of the rapes they knew about, feared or were exposed to in their communities.

In all sites, families were poor and there were high levels of unemployment among parents. In Tanzania about a quarter of parents were formally employed. Most were self-employed, working in jobs such as watchmen, petty traders or food vendors. This poverty affected schools, as the assistant head teacher in School A, Tanzania, notes:

> Some children come to school without breakfast or lunch. We have the tendency of donating uniforms for orphans…Some ask for money to buy the food.

In South Africa unemployment in both communities ranged from about 40 to 60 per cent, with many people caught in a cycle of low-paid or informal work. In Kenya, unemployment levels were similar to those observed in Cape Town. Similarly, adults in the urban communities were either unemployed or employed in temporary or low-paid jobs, such as security guards, gardeners, petty traders, food vendors or domestic workers.

Unemployment was frequently linked to substance abuse. Children frequently reported and pointed out youths, parents and other adults selling drugs in the community. Because of the high level of unemployment in the Cape Town and Mombasa sites, adults and youths were seen congregating on street corners; many would go to local taverns or shebeens (places selling alcohol without a licence) for illegal brew (known as *mnazi* in Mombasa) and to smoke marijuana. The Cape Town site reported greater hard-drug use, such as heroin, mandrax (methaqualone), tik (methamphetamine) and cocaine.

Availability of recreational spaces for children

Not surprisingly, in these communities recreational spaces for children were limited. In Cape Town the coloured community in which school B was located had a large, open, grassed park with a lone roundabout in the centre and a tarred space for playing basketball (but with no hoops). In the black community surrounding school A there were no parks nearby, although the school did have a soccer field. In the informal settlement in which most of the children lived there were just dusty roads that became muddy and potholed during the winter rainfall months.

In Tanzania muddy roads for rolling tyres, gnarled trees in compound courtyards and crumbling buildings to sit among and play cards were places for children's recreation. In Kenya, especially rural Mombasa, although there were wide-open spaces, there were few activities for children, and the nearby rubbish dump was both a source of recreation and survival for children.

Cultural and religious practices

With regard to ethnicities, in the South African township children in School A were predominantly black and spoke isiXhosa in addition to English. Children from School B in the coloured community spoke either English or Afrikaans as a home language, although School B's medium of instruction was English. This separateness mirrors South Africa's Apartheid history and remains common in impoverished areas. Only in suburban schools are there higher levels of 'racial' integration. In the black community in the study most young people professed Christianity, although some came from families that practised traditional African religion or both together. In the coloured community children came from Christian and Muslim families.

In Tanzania and Kenya most school communities were made up of a mixture of ethnicities, except in rural Mombasa where the tribe was predominantly Mijikenda. There was a mixture of Christian and Muslim students across the Tanzanian and Kenyan sites, with somewhat more Christian students in the Kenyan sites and somewhat more Muslim students in the Tanzanian sites. In all three countries there were strong traditional cultural practices in operation. In Dar es Salaam the area was dominated by people who had come from the coastal and southern parts of Tanzania, such as Wazaramu, Wandengereko, Wamatumbwi and Wamakonde. These dominant tribes have systematic ways of teaching their young people about sexual education, especially through the coming-of-age ceremony known as *Unyago*. This is also the case for the amaXhosa in Cape Town: the boys undergo an extended initiation (*umwaluko*) into adulthood, including a circumcision ritual, and both sexes are taught about their roles as adults by traditional teachers.

School resources, attendance and feeding schemes

The rapid ethnography also enabled us to observe the resources available in each school and country context. Though all schools were in impoverished environments, they had different levels of resources. School A in Cape Town was by far the best equipped. It had a library, hall, reception area, tuck shop, staffroom and storeroom. Most rooms had burglar bars over the windows and doors, and there was even a CCTV camera in the administration office. School B had large spaces, but not as much equipment. School A was in total contrast to the three schools in Mombasa, which had neither a hall nor a functioning library, and there was no burglar-proofing because of limited resources. In School A, Kenya, the library had been converted into a storeroom for sacks of maize for the feeding programme. In Dar es Salaam one school had a computer room. Two schools in Mombasa had defunct computer rooms. Schools B and C in Mombasa and one school in Dar es Salaam had no fences, and it was easy for the pupils to walk in and out of school. In Cape Town, both schools supported pupils by providing soccer kits and transport to local sports stadiums for competitions. However, in Mombasa, the situation was different and pupils participated in sports in their school uniforms and barefoot; in Tanzania there were very few sports activities.

A further marker of poverty was evidenced by school feeding schemes. In Cape Town and Mombasa all four schools had a free school feeding programme (see Photo 2). The feeding programmes acted as a pull factor for children to attend school, as they were sure to have a meal. For some, this was the only meal of the day because of the poverty at home. In Mombasa they were served githeri (boiled maize and beans/peas); in Cape Town they ate rice and soya soup. In all schools, a small fee was charged for the labour of cooking and fuel (five Kenyan shillings per meal in Mombasa and 50 cents in Cape Town). At both sites, children who failed to make the daily payment were sent home or punished in some way. Therefore, paradoxically, an intervention designed to enhance retention and participation in schools at times caused absenteeism if the child had to be sent home for food money. Tanzania did not have a feeding programme and the researchers reported that some children came to school with nothing to eat. Another factor that kept children in schools in Cape Town was that school attendance was a precondition to receiving a child support grant from the Department of Social Development. In some households, this was the only source of income.

The impact of HIV/AIDS on communities

In all three countries, participants identified HIV/AIDS as a problem in their communities. It was reported that there were many people in the communities living with HIV/AIDS and they kept their status to themselves until they became noticeably ill. Even in death AIDS was seldom spoken of as the cause. Once someone dies, rumours frequently circulate regarding the cause of death as having been AIDS. In South Africa, a Grade 6 teacher said: 'We don't hear about learners who are HIV-positive in the school.' However, others said there were many people in the community living with HIV/AIDS, but who tended to keep their status to themselves. Teachers in Mombasa and Dar es Salaam talked of children in their schools who were infected or whose parents were infected or had died, and so they were now orphans. In one Tanzanian school the assistant head teacher told the researcher that in the school there were three children who were directly affected by HIV/AIDS.

This brief report provided by the rapid ethnography highlights a central issue: the importance of social context through direct observations. The characteristics of the context influence the processes of teaching, learning and managing behaviour in school, and these become clearly evident in the next section. Poverty is visible in different forms and to different extents, materially and educationally, in each of these contexts. These contexts impact on the degree to which HIV/AIDS education is challenged – a topic to which we now turn.

The school as a context for HIV/AIDS education

So what did we learn about the schools and classrooms as a context for HIV/AIDS education? We knew from previous research already mentioned that schools exert a great influence on pupils' learning in the countries in which we researched (Ackers & Hardman 2001; Hardman et al. 2008; Scheerens 2000; Verspoor 2003). Other studies have also emphasised the importance of focusing on the nature of classroom pedagogy and on the school as a context for learning. In this section we focus on the physical nature of the school and classrooms, as well as the pedagogical practices observed within the classrooms. What did these observations show us in relation to our research questions about the primary sources and contents of sexual knowledges for young people in sub-Saharan Africa? How do they differ in terms of content and process of acquisition? And how do they interact with AIDS education received in the classroom?

Photos 3 to 5 show typical classrooms in each country. These pictures are fairly typical of schools in public-school systems in these three countries, and this is supported by our observations. There were differences in resource levels between the South African schools and those in Kenya and Tanzania. The South African schools had more and better-quality physical resources, such as basic equipment, like desks, chairs – and fewer learners per chair/bench – and books. These differences are explored further in the following sections. Details regarding student numbers and basic data about the schools are to be found in Tables 2.2 and 2.3 in Chapter 2.

Pedagogy

In using the word 'pedagogy' we imply something wider than classroom interaction. We are focusing on all the activities of educating young people – the principles, beliefs and practices in classrooms, including classroom interactions. Hardman et al. (2008: 56) show that 'there is a paucity of data in sub-Saharan Africa generally into how teachers actually teach in the classroom'. However, available research from across the continent indicates a high prevalence of teacher-centred, authoritarian and didactic pedagogies (Altinyelken 2010; Chisholm & Leyendecker 2008; O'Sullivan 2004; Vavrus 2009). A synthesis of research on pedagogy in Africa concluded that 'undesirable practices' persisted, which could be described as follows:

> This kind of teaching is generally labeled 'traditional'. It can be described in a nutshell as rigid, chalk-and-talk, teacher-centered/dominated, lecture-driven. It is reported to place students in a passive role and to limit their activity in class to memorizing facts and reciting them back to the teacher…The kind of teaching thus described…is reported to foster only lower order skills. It is said to exemplify the teaching/transmission paradigm as opposed to that of learning. (Dembele & Lefoka, 2007: 535)

Our rapid ethnography does not claim to be an in-depth study of classroom behaviour or teaching and learning practices, but it is a detailed snapshot and seems to be in accord with other studies (although limited in number) on pedagogy in sub-Saharan classrooms. Some of these studies include Kenya (Ackers & Hardman 2001; Bunyi 1997; Pontefract & Hardman 2005); Tanzania (O-saki & Agu 2002); and South Africa (Chick 1996). In exploring pedagogy through observation in classrooms we focused on identifying modes of learning and teaching, teacher-pupil relationships and interactions, as well as assumptions concerning power, authority and control. We did so in order to hypothesise about understandings and theories of teaching and learning in action, since each of these features of pedagogy impinges on knowledge acquisition and knowledge legitimisation.

Teacher-pupil relationships

In keeping with the literature described above, in most of the schools in which we worked, the teachers' style of relating to pupils was largely authoritative. Processes in the classroom were teacher-led and teacher-initiated. This is in keeping with African respect for tradition and authority (Prophet & Rowell 1993), which was more dominant in Kenya and Tanzania in this study. For example, teachers expected pupils to clean the chalkboards and tidy classrooms, and nominated pupils to act in various leadership positions. In Kenya and Tanzania the teachers carried canes, and corporal punishment was acceptable and used. However, in Kenya and Tanzania the atmosphere between pupils and teachers was also supportive, and we observed the use of humour and sharing of jokes. Children were observed walking with teachers, chatting animatedly and sharing peanuts. In Kenya teachers were observed supporting pupils and creating rapport with them. Some did this by clapping and asking students for responses to what were established rituals and banter. For example, in Kenya a female maths teacher invited the class to 'let us clap for her with flowers', a term pupils understood to mean clapping and shaking hands. She then asked the class: 'What colour is the flower?', to which a number of pupils replied 'red and pink like her skirt'. The warmth, respect and familiarity between pupils and teachers were plain to see in this exchange. Teaching and learning facilitated through the use of humour can be seen in this example from School B in Kenya:

Female maths teacher:	Are they mangoes, avocados?
Pupils:	No, they are minutes.
Female maths teacher:	Then you must label.

In Kenya, teachers also used local idioms to admonish students, such as a Swahili teacher who told a student, 'Ameharibu mchuzi huyu' (she has ruined the stew).

In South African classrooms, while interactive learning was visible at times, there were also numerous examples of disruptive behaviour by pupils in the classroom. In School B a small group of boys frequently misbehaved and the class teacher spent an inordinate amount of time dealing with them and trying to regain the class's attention. This severely limited the amount of teaching and learning that could take place in the class. It was also clear that this was not uncommon. Researchers observed low-level disruption or misbehaviour behind teachers' backs when they were writing on the chalkboard. In some classrooms teachers did not turn up for class or were very late, and this too appeared not to be unusual. In School A the pupils sat in same-sex groups.

A further observation concerned the extent to which teachers lived in the communities in which they taught. This varied in the three sites, although teachers tended not to live in the communities in which they taught. Teachers at School B in South Africa and School A in rural Mombasa are notable exceptions. Those in urban Mombasa, Dar es Salaam and School A, Cape Town, lived elsewhere in more affluent neighbourhoods. Therefore, teachers represented a higher social class in the schools. This too might be a phenomenon worthy of further investigation with regard to teaching and learning in the classroom.

Teaching and learning in the classroom

The observed learning and teaching model, apart from one case, was a didactic teacher-led style. The pattern was largely initiation-response-follow-up. There was much lifting of hands for answering questions and for marking of work. Pupils would chorus answers to questions and sometimes the teacher would pick pupils by name. When the teachers taught much time was spent facing the chalkboard, writing notes for the children to copy. Sometimes pupils were invited to work out a problem on the board. One female Swahili teacher in Kenya responded to a female pupil's request for help in solving a problem on the chalkboard by saying: 'You tell us. I'm the student now.'

In South Africa, since the advent of democracy there have been intentional efforts by the National Department of Education to ensure that learning is group-based, continuously assessed and as interactive as possible. This outcomes-based education approach was especially disliked by teachers in School A, who said it was connected to the children's misbehaviour in the classroom.

It was noted that in many cases, pupils – and some teachers – were not very confident about their own knowledge. The book was seen as the source of knowledge and there was great dependence on textbooks. Pupils would be asked to close the books first, think and not just go straight to the answers in the book. However, there was little sign of independent learning strategies, such as taking notes while the teacher taught. This ties in with Tabulawa's (1997) research in Botswana, which also found heavy reliance on the textbook as a primary source of knowledge. After exploring the reasons for this through in-depth interviews, Tabulawa concluded that the pupils and teachers both saw the primary purpose of education as memorising the facts required to pass the exams, which, in turn, led to the possibility of well-paid employment. Similarly, Vavrus's (2009) research at a teacher training college in Tanzania found that trainee teachers did not see the purpose of facilitating broader discussion about the novels on the literature syllabus because the time could be more effectively spent learning facts in preparation for the national exam. This may explain why the textbook, as the carrier of these required facts, would be accorded such high status.

As has already been discussed, the physical resources available to each school and in the countries varied considerably. Some classrooms were equipped with sufficient books and handouts for each pupil; in others books were shared between classes, and teachers' notes on the chalkboard served as the only source of information. In a number of schools there was no soundproofing between classrooms and pupils came into lessons to borrow basic equipment, whereas in School A in South Africa there was a fully equipped audio-visual centre with a television and other items. The availability of these physical resources clearly had an influence on the teaching and learning approaches adopted.

Again, our findings fit with those of the studies cited earlier (e.g. Ackers & Hardman 2001; Bunyi 1997; Chick 1996; Hardman et al. 2008), which also portray a teacher-led, lengthy recitation and explanation style of pedagogy, with pupils largely remaining passive. The study in Nigeria by Hardman et al. (2008) revealed a pattern of teacher exposition taking up most of the lesson (70 per cent) and with questions being largely ritualistic and closed (98 per cent). Questions, which might be considered an active teaching method, were the most common strategy used to elicit student responses. Although questions might have been used to expand learning by promoting critical reflection, they were instead largely employed to control and engage. Choral responses were common, and in our observations when a teacher asked a question and there was an answer, in 58 per cent of the cases there was no further follow-up. This pattern of interaction was common in all three of the countries.

Although Tanzania, Kenya and South Africa have all endorsed interactive, learner-centred pedagogies at the policy level, the patterns of interaction observed are still not surprising. Research in countries that have made concerted efforts to move towards more interactive, learner-centred pedagogies, such as South Africa (Nykiel-Herbert 2004) and Uganda (Altinyelken 2010), found that while the new policies led to an increase in teachers' asking questions of students, these questions remained closed and limited to basic information recall. This demonstrates the difficulty of moving beyond traditional pedagogical approaches in the classroom. Both Nykiel-Herbert (2004) and Altinyelken (2010) conclude that instigating more substantive changes in classroom interaction is challenging because it is not only barriers of inadequate resources and training that need to be overcome, but also an incongruence between these approaches and teachers' views on the nature of knowledge, the purpose of education and the desired relationships between adults and children. Al-Hinai (2007: 46) somewhat more optimistically argues that 'educational practices which focus on rote learning and teacher centred approaches stem from a lack of expertise and sometimes a lack of means rather than from cultural restriction'. This important differentiation is one to which we will repeatedly return.

Orphaned and vulnerable children in school

In all sites there were orphaned and vulnerable children. For example, School A in Dar es Salaam identified three such children. Of these, one pupil now had TB. His parents had died of AIDS-related illness and he now lived with his grandmother. In Schhol B in Cape Town, one lived only with her father. Her parents had separated and her mother remarried. This new husband had subsequently died the previous year from an AIDS-related illness, and her mother was now living with HIV and on treatment. This shows that HIV/AIDS was a personal problem in the lives and homes of the school community.

A school in Mombasa had a total of 36 orphaned and vulnerable children. In response to these children's needs, the school had organised a feeding programme specifically for this group of young people, with well-wishers from the community contributing the food and money needed. A particular wealthy community member was the key donor and personally made sure that there was food for these children. However, the researcher at one point witnessed a parent, who was also a member of the school board, chastising the deputy head teacher for not making sure that all the orphaned and vulnerable children were fed at school. The teacher said in reply that it was because some infected children lacked appetite and refused to eat. Clearly, this parent saw teachers' roles as going beyond teaching and the classroom, and extending to nurturing.

Engaging in HIV-related education

In the Mombasa and Cape Town schools, there was evidence that teachers engaged in HIV/AIDS education. In Dar es Salaam, however, researchers reported that though the pupils seemed to want to know about HIV/AIDS, it was not taught. A Muslim teacher said that he did not teach anything to do with the topic because 'it is not said in the curriculum'. He did, however, report that he asked Grades 5/6/7 to stay back once a month and talked to them about the dangers of 'drinking and smoking' and how to keep away from 'bad social habits'. Some teachers in this school also said that if there was a curriculum that specified it and extra money to pay them, they would teach HIV/AIDS education after normal school hours. A number of teachers expressed the view that they did not need to teach about HIV/AIDS, since it formed part of 'reproduction' and 'sexually transmitted diseases', which were taught in science/biology and in life-skills lessons. Notably, School C in Dar es Salaam was involved in an HIV/AIDS education programme through the international NGO Africa Medical and Research Foundation.

In all three Mombasa schools, the teachers infused HIV/AIDS information into the subjects they taught. This was particularly possible for Swahili, maths and Christian religious education, and happened in 4 out of the 48 lessons observed by the researcher. For example, a male maths teacher used the following exercise: 'A hospital had 35 inpatients tested for HIV. Ten per cent of these were HIV-negative. How many were HIV-positive?'

Notably, some teachers were also more open than others on sexual matters. They encouraged pupils to speak up and be open. If pupils were too shy to speak, the teacher gave the answer or said the words that the pupils were too bashful to use, such as 'condoms' and 'vaginal discharge'. This is illustrated in the following exchange between two male teachers, one of Swahili, who was also the head teacher, and the other a teacher of Christian religious education (CRE), and a mixed-sex group of pupils:

Swahili teacher:	How do you get AIDS?
Pupils:	Sex, giving a kiss, blood transfusion, breast milk.
Swahili teacher:	[Acts out the kiss and the class laughs.]
CRE teacher:	Where is the virus found in the body?
Pupils:	Blood, saliva, semen.
CRE teacher:	Where else? [Silence] I know you know. You are just shy to say it. [Silence] Vaginal fluids [he translates for them into Swahili] *yale maji maji yanayotoka katika kile kitendo* [the fluids discharged by the woman during that activity].
Swahili teacher:	But how can you protect yourself?
Boy:	Don't have sex *kiholelaholela*.
Swahili teacher:	But if I have a wife I should not make love to her? [Laughter].
Pupils:	Nooooooo –
Swahili teacher:	Some make love when they are not married...so what should they do? [Silence] I know you know. [More silence] For those who can't wait we say you use condoms. But it's better for adults. For you we say wait for marriage.
Pupils:	Yes.

Despite this attempted openness by teachers, it is interesting to note that even the teacher avoids the term 'sex' when translating from Swahili into English and instead says 'during that activity'.

In School B, Cape Town, one teacher who was responsible for HIV/AIDS education did not mention the word 'sex' at all in her teaching. Instead, she frequently said 'do their thing' when referring to intercourse. When prodded by the researcher as to why she used a euphemism, she said she deliberately did not use the word 'sex' because pupils ended up telling their parents what the teacher had said in class and they, in turn, would blame the teacher for talking about sex to their children. This presents a dilemma whereby the teachers who are meant to teach and be agents of change are limited and influenced by sociocultural contexts. This teacher felt that she had been effective in an HIV/AIDS education lesson when learners gave the correct answers about HIV/AIDS. She saw this as proof that they have gained knowledge. However, we now know that information does not necessarily lead to behaviour change, and a grasp of knowledge alone is not effective in HIV/AIDS prevention. This teacher's teaching design also involved her sharing her personal experiences of being married and role playing. However, the researcher observed that role playing in an HIV/AIDS education class led to jibes and labelling. For example, a boy who had been used in the role play for HIV transmission was later nicknamed 'Virus'. This caused the boy to become worried and he asked the researcher if he was now infected. She explained that the teacher was using them to make it easier for the children to understand how HIV can be spread from one person to another. This school also held an AIDS candlelight, a special assembly where the theme for the day was to remember those who were sick with HIV/AIDS, and those who had died from the disease. The researcher wondered if these were indeed routine practices or due to her research focus.

The concept of fear and believing in fate also emerged. A number of children expressed the belief that it was impossible to protect oneself from HIV/AIDS. For some, HIV/AIDS was seen as a condition that is to be feared, and is shrouded in silence and myths. As a result, pupils exhibited a sense of helplessness when asked about it – as evidenced by the following words (strongly disputed by the teacher), spoken by a boy in School A, Kenya:

> But, teacher, if you have an accident on a bus your blood can mix. That's why I'm telling you, you cannot protect yourself from AIDS. Even when you don't want it, it finds you.

Clearly, teaching and learning about HIV and AIDS in a primary school-classroom is a complex under-taking, fraught with hazards that have to be carefully navigated. These hazards include pedagogical styles, fear of parents' reactions, children's concrete understandings, cultural and social taboos and the availability of physical resources to aid teaching and learning.

Reflections on knowledge, power and pedagogy

The pictures painted above of the school environment and social context fit with other research studies on pedagogy. All show that the model of learning employed in most of the observed classrooms was heavily teacher-dependent and one in which the notion of knowledge as residing within the book was also visible. This problematises the notion of whether pupils could act as legitimate sources of knowledge and whether they would be able to interrogate and analyse how the origin of their knowledge might affect the message they received from it. Furthermore, in our observations, pupils' everyday knowledge did not seem to feature in the classrooms. Many sexuality and HIV/AIDS education programmes – and this research study – are premised on models of social-constructivist theories of active learning, and involve engaging with pupils' everyday knowledge. By contrast, the model of learning and behaviour change embedded in the practices that our researchers observed was one that was based on a transmission model and a view that giving information is the prime lever for behaviour change.

The other issue of interest relates to notions of children and their sexuality, and the place of sexuality in school. In the observations it is possible to detect different positionings of pupils and models of the ideal pupil. Here we draw on the work of Allen (2007) in New Zealand. She alerts us to the notion of competing discourses within schools and contradictory processes, as Bernstein (1990a) argued. On the one hand, school stakeholders (i.e. parents, teachers and community leaders) are almost always agreed, especially in the contexts which we describe, that abstinence is the primary message for children and youth, and sex as desire is seldom spoken of in formal teaching within school contexts. On the other hand, HIV/AIDS education is premised upon the notion that young people are sexual beings and sexually active, and that young people should engage in safe sex when they are sexually active. These discourses of prohibition and protection are contradictory – and yet due to the AIDS pandemic now exist alongside each other in the school context. These protective and prohibitive discourses also raise further questions. Do teachers and schools see young people as having sexual agency or a voice on sexual matters? Do adults conceive of young people as sexual beings? In all our primary schools, in all three country sites, we observed indications of sexualised behaviour and sexual activity. Nevertheless, there remains evidence of much ambivalence regarding the nature of children's sexuality from adults in our preliminary data. The ambivalence seems to apply also to the idea of whether sexuality education should be provided at all, and some uncertainty about whether it will make matters better or worse.

These observations also connect with the position adopted by the schools in relation to the community, especially with regard to sex and HIV/AIDS education. Again, we saw different positions being adopted. In some cases, the schools perceived their role to be that of change agents leading the way in giving a widely conceived education on HIV/AIDS. In other cases, schools saw themselves as reflections of community attitudes, in other words, the status quo, and were fearful of challenging them. In some schools there was high visibility and some autonomy in the development of HIV/AIDS work. In others it was not visible, often absent and teachers awaited instructions, sometimes fearfully or belligerently. The rapid ethnographies provided a useful backdrop against which to explore the more in-depth findings gained from the detailed consultations and interviews with pupils and teachers. They also helped to link what our participants said to what we saw.

The final reflection concerns the complexity of the position of teachers in these schools. There is clearly a connection between the ambivalences in the community around sexuality and sex education and teachers' behaviour in schools. There were instances in our observation when teachers spoke of their concern about a clash between their views and those of community members. If we add to this the everyday difficulty of teaching on this controversial and personal topic, something that challenges teachers all over the world, then we see that the task is complex indeed.

The research studies cited in this chapter have highlighted the lack of preparation and confidence of teachers in primary schools[9] in these three countries. The controlling and lecture-type discourses and patterns of interaction seem to arise from a lack of theory, reflection on practice and preparation. The rapid expansion of primary education and the shortage of resources have had an impact on the quality of teacher education, especially initial teacher education. Two important questions arise for educational developers: what sort of support would teachers need to engage in effective interactive HIV/AIDS education, and what can aid teachers in the perceived clash of expectations between their community and their classroom? These are two key questions with which we have begun to engage and to which we will return in the final chapter.

---

9   Helleve et al. (2009a) provide evidence that teachers in South Africa and Tanzania at the secondary level reported being confident in teaching sex education. However, this was not the case for the primary-school teachers whom the researchers observed in the present study.

CHAPTER 5

Young people's in and out of school sexual knowledges

Everyone knows that 'children have no sex', which is why they are forbidden to talk about it, why one closes one's eyes and stops one's ears whenever they show evidence to the contrary. (Foucault 1976: 4)

Exclusion occurs because of an unwarranted disparity between curricular content and the sensuous content of everyday lives of the children…this disparity constitutes an unnecessary barrier to the learners; it is a barrier arbitrarily constructed by agents of the status quo and it must therefore be removed in the interests of empowerment and emancipation. (Taylor 2000: 70)

This chapter answers the first of our research questions: what are the primary *sources* and *contents* of sexual knowledges for young people in sub-Saharan Africa, and how do these knowledges differ in terms of content and process of acquisition? In addressing this question, our research takes Foucault and Taylor's assertions seriously. In what ways are children's lives sexualised and how much do they know or want to know about the intimacies and mechanics of sex? And furthermore, how closely aligned or how far apart are young people's everyday sexual knowledges from the knowledge they receive at school?

Methods and theories

The data presented here are derived from the photovoice method described in Chapter 2. According to Wang and Burris (1994, 1997), photovoice is a production of knowledge through photography. It puts cameras in the hands of the local community – people such as children, rural women and grassroots' workers, who normally have little access to those people who make decisions over their lives – and it allows them to speak through images. This is an especially powerful methodology when working with those who are marginalised or who might find it difficult to articulate their answers through other means, such as interviews. Children are, therefore, ideal candidates for photovoice because it helps them describe their lives and experiences in the absence of advanced verbal ability.

In this study, we gave pupils cameras to capture the sources and content of their sexual knowledges from the two worlds that they predominantly occupy – the school and the community. Trusting them with the camera gave them the power to produce knowledge, sustained their interest in the construction of knowledge and provided us with an image of their lives both in and out of school. The pupils got 'the freedom to pick and choose the people…[and objects] who are important…It is this immense freedom which the camera gives to participants which distinguishes it from traditional paper and pencil tests' (Jones 2004: 190). The photos taken acted as an entry point to a non-self-conscious discussion of their sexual knowledges and worlds in and out of school.

Bernstein's (1971) theory of knowledge was helpful in understanding the role and implications of knowledges from these two worlds – in school and out of school. He calls the knowledge learnt from school vertical, or hierarchical, knowledge, which is based on theory and abstract principles, and is assessed. Knowledge acquired out of school is horizontal, or everyday knowledge, which is context-dependent (Scott 2008). As presented in Chapter 1, when it comes to HIV/AIDS education, the formal, or vertical, knowledge offered often does not meet the needs of young people because it fails to include the sociocultural aspects of their everyday lives and everyday knowledges. This autonomy of, and boundary between, knowledge from the two worlds may lead to exclusion, as Taylor (2000: 70) states in the extract above, 'A barrier arbitrarily constructed by agents of the status quo'. In this present study these 'agents' would be parents, teachers and other stakeholders, including curriculum developers (all of whom are adults). As will be seen in this chapter, pupils are offered little or no control over the selection and organisation of the content and pedagogy of the sex and HIV/AIDS education they receive. An abstinence-only curriculum impresses upon children that sex is only for marriage, ignores the sexual world that young people are already engaging in and presents them as asexual, childlike, innocent and dependent on adults for guidance and protection (Allen 2007; Bhana 2007b, 2007c; Campbell 2003; Kirby 2002). This is a far cry from what children see, know and are doing, as will be presented next.

In everyday terms, we wanted to find out what children know about sex and AIDS, and where they learn this information. We now present the data derived from our pupils on *where* they acquired their sexual knowledges (sources) and *what* messages were acquired (content). The out-of-school sexual knowledges are presented first followed by the in-school knowledges. We conclude by comparing how these two sources of knowledge differ and discuss how pupils' sexual knowledges are affected by their sociocultural contexts.

Out-of-school sources and content of sexual knowledges

After analysing children's photographs and the interviews that accompanied them, a number of main themes emerged regarding children's everyday sources of sexual knowledge. These were seeing sexual intercourse in the streets and open spaces, including transactional sex; observing and experiencing sexual exploitation and abuse in the streets and home; gaining formal and incidental learning from parents and other social institutions, and practical sexual learning from neighbourhood peers.

Seeing sexual intercourse in the streets and open spaces

In Chapter 4 we described the kind of environment in which our pupils lived (see Photos 6 and 7). Though resources in contexts varied among the three countries, common to all were that the neighbourhoods were poor with limited sanitation systems and overcrowded homes; pupils reported that they were from single-parent homes; and they lived in communities where people visibly abused drugs, had commercial sex and sex for pleasure, practised crime and lived with HIV/AIDS. Pupils reported that some young people whiled away their time gambling, playing pool, darts and draughts, and engaged in sex and substance abuse (see Photos 8 and 9). Campbell (2003) in her study in informal settlements in South Africa described these as not only forms of recreation, but escapism from the frustrations of poverty.

Kustiantu from Kenya aptly sums up what most of the pupils in the three countries thought of their environments:

> My environment is bad, people engage in drinking all the time. There are people who give children hard drugs to make them survive and push on the day. Some children roam around, some are not in school, and some have dropped out of school. People engage in sex anyhow (unprotected and often). It is easy to be lured into sex…there is no one to tell us [teach us] a positive thing about sex and HIV/AIDS. (Kustiantu, boy, aged 12, School C, Kenya)

In the neighbourhoods there were numerous beer dens, or shebeens; some pupils reporting living next door to them or having parents or landlords who ran these taverns. Some homes doubled up as beer dens. Activities within these places, or activities that happened as a consequence of people visiting them were an influential source of sexual knowledges. Four pupils (Zuhara, a 12-year-old girl from School B, Tanzania; Chileza, a 12-year-old boy from School A, South Africa; Binti, a 12-year-old girl from School C, Kenya; and Gatete, a 17-year-old boy from School C, Kenya) said that the drinking places in their areas increased uninhibited sexual behaviour and they linked this to the spread of HIV/AIDS. In these neighbourhoods, drug abuse was also 'common, extremely common', as Binti put it. Binti's family had rented a room within 10 attached single-roomed houses, and not only did the landlady use one of the rooms as a beer den and brothel, but her adult son also sold and smoked *bhang* (marijuana). Photo 10 shows him and his friend slumped (and 'high') against a wall outside Binti's home. Maria is a 13-year-old girl from School C, Kenya. Photo 11 shows a male youth passed out outside Maria's gate. Photo 12 shows a similar scene, but this time with a child clearly visible in the picture.

However, children not only reported what they saw in their immediate environment, but also spoke of their peers' behaviour. Some pupils were reported to smoke cigarettes and cannabis in a hookah (water pipe). Anna, a 12-year-old girl from School B, South Africa, talking about her classmates, said: 'Like, Britney, she started out smoking the hookah pipe but now she is doing tik [crystal methamphetamine], dagga [marijuana] and cigarettes. Kylie in our class also smokes almost every day.' These 'leisure activities' sometimes exacerbated truancy, as reported by pupils and teachers.

A number of children made the connection between substance abuse and sex. Binti explained how her mum tried to shield her from seeing drunkards having sex, and how she had learnt foul language from them, such as 'your mother's vagina' and 'you prostitute'. Similarly, Juma, a 12-year-old boy from School A in Tanzania, explained how smoking marijuana had made youths in his village 'get euphoric effects which led them into doing sex'. Binti and Dalila had seen sexual intercourse live in the public spaces of their neighbourhood as a result of drug intoxication:

> When they inhale these substances…they don't wait to get a room, they get any man and start having sex in public…there and then, at the point of contact…I see them…outside our house… in the football field. Especially on Saturday and Sunday the field is packed. The prostitutes, the drunkards…it means the children know what sex is because they see it. (Binti, girl, aged 12, School C, Kenya)

> It is the norm to make love in the open…even as cars pass by. They do it there and then. They do not go to hidden places, they do not fear…they have drunk and used drugs, they will not care who sees them. (Dalila, girl, aged 13, School C, Kenya)

Kustiantu from Kenya also described how on Sundays, 'the golden boys', a gang of about 30 male youths, took over some classrooms in a school in his neighbourhood and had group sex, leaving the school littered with used condoms and faeces. He also told of having seen some of the gang members masturbate in the open, and of witnessing adults fondling each other in the presence of young children, as shown in Photo 13. Kustiantu told the researcher what he had previously seen, 'With one hand this man was distracting the child with a telephone…With the other hand, he was touching this woman somewhere under her dress between the thighs.'

This is a good example of how perceptive children are despite parents' efforts to shield them from sexual issues. It is possible too that the child being distracted could be aware of what the adults are up to, and if not, the likelihood is high that he will soon come to understand. Photo 13 is also a good example of the profound nature of photovoice, whereby a simple photo such as this holds a deeper and complex message.

Pupils' photographs also revealed their awareness of same-sex relationships. In Kenya, they had seen gay couples (both male and female) particularly on the beach – a cosmopolitan meeting place between locals and tourists. Dalila took pictures of a young lesbian couple and was able to follow them into an alley where they allowed her to watch as they fondled each other. 'I saw them touching each other…I asked if I could take their photo and they allowed me…they were touching each other's breasts…and unzipping their skirts,' said Dalila. However, it was clear in all three countries that same-sex relationships were not approved of. Zama, a 12-year-old girl from School A in South Africa, said that 'gays are not supposed to have sex because they are both male'. Achieng (aged 14) and Dalila (aged 12), both girls from School C, Kenya, said that homosexuals in their neighbourhoods were often beaten and assaulted, 'The community sees them [homosexuals] as idiots.' These comments by children illustrate Foucault's (1976) analysis of the social control or regulation of sexuality, in this case, with regard to choice of sexual partners.

Pupils also reported incidences of incest within the family. In South Africa, 12-year-old Trevor from School B spoke about how one family member had infected others with HIV/AIDS: 'He got it and he spread [it], almost the whole family got it because…Everyone had sex with the cousin, and a cousin, and a cousin.' The examples above of children's exposure to 'live sex' demonstrate that the social control, rules and regulations surrounding sex are limited in poor communities in the absence of privacy, sobriety, safety and adequate material resources. In the same vein, exposure to progressive norms, such as the acceptance of homosexual relationships, is frequently absent, largely due to a lack of exposure and little education with regard to human rights.

Transactional sex in the neighbourhood

In all three countries, pupils were aware of the exchange of sex for money. In South Africa, Anna (School B) reported that sex was sold for as little as 50 cents in her neighbourhood. Fathiya, a 12-year-old girl from School A, Kenya, summed it up well: 'When there is no food at home because of drought, a man will give you money and you will accept.' Hakika, a 12-year-old girl from School B, Tanzania, added, 'You have expenses at home, life is hard. Maybe you don't have examination fees.' Campbell (2003: 63) describes this as 'gift sex' and argues that it is not shrouded in the shame and stigma associated with prostitution, but is seen as a means of survival. Tatu, a 12-year-old girl from School A in Tanzania, said that there was a guest house and bar near her home 'where female children wear short outfits and dance, and when a man comes, he takes one of them to a guest house'.

Arguably, the expectation of youth in this environment to practise abstinence is more difficult and frequently far removed from the reality of their daily lives. Instead, the prevailing information they learn in their community is that sex can be one way of earning a living. Sex also provided status, a sense of maturity and feelings of power. Sandi, a 13-year-old boy from School A in South Africa, observed: 'When you are 13, you can be attracted to an older person as a boyfriend, one who is already circumcised,[10] who has a car, money and is famous.' Achieng, a 14-year-old girl from School C in Kenya, said that girls in Mombasa were attracted to the white male tourists who frequented the beach.

She illustrated the scenario of sex for money at the beach by assembling her dolls (see Photo 14) and giving them roles – a white male tourist with two schoolgirls. Jewkes et al. (2005) show that although such relationships are not condoned by society, they could be privately accepted, encouraged and seen as advantageous in poorer households. They further argue that female peers may be envious of those involved in sexual relationships because of the gifts they get. Girls involved may also be described as exhibiting 'pride in the fruits of demonstrations of sexuality' (Jewkes et al. 2005: 1812) for their ability to contribute income to a household and enhance their own status.

10   In some communities, only circumcised men are seen as adult. An uncircumcised man would be viewed as a 'boy'.

In some instances, these intergenerational relationships evolved into a long-term relationship and/or marriage. Fathiya (12-year-old girl, School A, Kenya) explained how a girl from her school had dropped out to marry an older man and had six children with him. There was also a class-6 boy who had met a married woman at the local disco and had consequently dropped out of school to live with her. In Tanzania, 12-year-old Nyambui explained how so-called sugar mommies at a local brothel targeted boys his age:

> There are old women who sell themselves at brothels…so when the youth want to practise sexual intercourse they go to these brothels. Some young [people] go there after finishing their jobs… and here everyone who comes with money gets in… Unfortunately there are youths as young as I who go to these old women…I have witnessed them many times…but let us say it is not good for youths to go to such a place. (Nyambui, boy, aged 12, School A, Tanzania)

Young people in our study provided evidence that in the communities in which they lived, transactional and intergenerational sex was practised by both sexes. The brothels and guest houses offered the place and opportunity for young people to 'taste' sex. For some pupils, sex for money happened in their own homes. Anna (School B, South Africa) told of a classmate's mother who was a drug addict and who slept with her own brother to get money.

Experiencing and observing sexual exploitation and abuse in the streets and home

Anna offered another reason for intergenerational sex that was far removed from poverty – although perhaps not so far removed from the ignorance that often accompanies poverty. This was the myth of sexual purity and sexual cleansing: 'Men think teenagers are not infected with this disease, so they sleep with them.' Wilton (1997) and others bear this out: 'Men are taking younger partners in an attempt to protect themselves from HIV infection' Wilton (1997: 56). The reasoning behind this is that because children are virgins, they are 'pure'. Sexual cleansing, an associated belief, may also have aggravated rape cases among children and babies, and increased child prostitution because men who are infected with HIV/AIDS rape them in an attempt to 'cleanse' themselves of the infection (Jewkes et al. 2005; Leclerc-Madlala 2002; Siringi 2002). Girls in this study were aware of and influenced by rape and sexual abuse in their communities. Nonthle (girl, aged 12, School B, South Africa) said, 'Nowadays we cannot walk about at night…there are gangsters and rapists.' In Kenya, Binti reported how a gang of boys who had smoked *bhang* had attacked her and her friend and further attempted to rape her friend:

> Just some days back…like 6 p.m. in the evening…we were on our way from Madrasa [religious school] and we ran into this gang of boys who were smoking bhang…One of them grabbed my friend and she fell, and they started to undress her…I ran into the neighbourhood and started screaming, and the boys ran away but they had already removed her clothes…These boys are bad…they cat-call when you pass near them and shout, 'come closer and see what we can do to you…we can baptise you' [insinuates having sex for the first time]. (Binti, girl, aged 12, School C, Kenya)

This incident highlights how unsafe the streets can be for girls. Jewkes et al. (2005) posit that female children are rendered especially vulnerable to abuse through a combination of dominant patriarchal ideology compounded by age hierarchies. In other words, men can take what they want and elders are beyond reproach. Bhana (2007b: 318) articulates the 'bad men discourse', a discourse evidenced by Binti as she recounted the attempted rape ('these boys are bad…they cat-call when you pass near them and shout, "come closer and see what we can do to you…we can baptise you"'). Bhana argues that the polarisation of gendered identities (a labelling adapted even in HIV/AIDS campaigns) presents boys as bad and as sexual predators, and girls as needing protection from dangerous forms of sexuality

(Bhana 2007c: 433). Boys seem to have taken up this labelling and showcase an unguarded sex drive, which Foucault (1976: 39) calls a 'Don Juan' sexuality that they cannot control. Foucault uses the story of Don Juan to metaphorically describe a man driven in spite of himself by the madness of sex. This has been used as an excuse for rape, where it is the woman's/girl's provocation that prompts rape. Some pupils in Kenya and South Africa said girls brought rape upon themselves if they dressed in a provocative or 'sexy way'. Jewkes et al. (2005: 1814) presented similar findings where teenage girls in South Africa who wore short skirts and trousers were judged to be deliberately taunting men. Men, in turn, viewed this 'provocation' as a dare and responded with rape, further entrenching their dominance:

> The idea of uncontrollable desire operated more pervasively as a discursive device to coerce girls into more conservative styles of dressing and behaviour, and to remind them of the need to respect (inherently dangerous) men. It could also be used to explain some rape as 'biological' rather than 'sociological', and thus absolve guilt. (Jewkes et al. 2005: 1814)

Therefore, even if girls know about the pleasurable side of sex (as discussed later in this chapter), their pleasure is overlaid by the material, cultural, gendered and social circumstances in their communities, factors which make them vulnerable to sexual abuse and prostitution (Bhana 2007b). Some girls talked about how homes were not safe either. Rifquah in South Africa reported how her friend Carol's grandfather displayed paedophilic behaviour:

> Carol's grandfather…the other day he told me that I should take a photo of my private parts and show him. He has also tried to ask Anna…So I said, 'I'm going to phone the police', so he walked away quickly. But the other day at church, he told me that I should go to his house. I told him I was going to tell my mother, so he did not insist…but I didn't tell my mother. (Rifquah, aged 12, School B, South Africa)

It can be argued that Rifquah did not tell her mother out of embarrassment of talking to her about a sexual issue. Alternatively, her silence may be due to cultural prohibitions based on mistaken notions of respect and how it relates to age and gender hierarchies, which often follow a patriarchal code. It is, therefore, easy to see how a child may not feel confident to report bad behaviour from an adult, especially a man. This is similar to a finding in Oluga et al. (2010), who state that children felt uncomfortable reporting sexual abuse to parents both for cultural reasons and because they felt they would not be believed and would be punished. From the evidence above, it is plausible to conclude that children (and girls in particular) are targets for sexual abuse within and outside the home. Their sexual knowledge, while including pleasure, is frequently overlaid with survival and fear. Therefore, understanding young people's sociocultural contexts as this study has done, gives us a better chance to position children's sexual knowledges and understandings within the sexual, cultural, material and social milieus of their communities.

Formal and incidental learning from parents

As well as seeing sex in their immediate environment, children also reported that parents were a primary source of sexual knowledge. Types of messages received from parents ranged from information about abstinence until marriage to using condoms for protection. Children reported various teaching styles from their parents. For example, parents in Tanzania were frequently reported as using a traditional oral narrative method often recounted by grandparents, whereby children would sit and listen to their words of wisdom (see Photos 15 and 16).

By contrast, a Xhosa pupil in South Africa said that parents and grandparents did not talk to children about HIV/AIDS not only because they were illiterate, but also because they themselves grew up in silence. Because of this, 12-year-old Lonwabo (School A) suggested that it was the children and youth who should educate parents 'so they can share the knowledge with their peers [other parents] because some of them do not want to talk about this disease…It's the way they were brought up and told it was a taboo to talk about AIDS.' Conversely, parents in Tanzania were described as reliable sources of counsel. Maimuna reported that her mother not only bought her books on HIV/AIDS, but also discussed them with her, especially on not sharing sharp objects. She concluded:

> Mother's teachings have given me confidence in making decisions concerning HIV/AIDS. I have learned what to do if I do not want to be infected. And if I am infected, what measures I have to take so as to survive. (Maimuna, girl, aged 12, School B, Tanzania)

Just like some of the South African parents, however, there was also a reticence on the part of this Tanzanian mother – Maimuna said her mother did not discuss relationships even when asked. This is a good example of parents giving only factual knowledge, but withholding information on sex and relationships. In Bhana's (2007b: 310) view, Maimuna's mother could be regulating knowledge about sexuality, thwarting sexual curiosity and upholding sexual innocence.

These are similar to the views of Allen (2007), Foucault (1976), Ingham (2005) and Kehily (2002). Bhana (2007c) and Aggleton and Campbell (2000) add that adults are free and open when talking about the facts of HIV/AIDS, but the converse is true when it came to talking about sex, which they construct as dangerous, something to be feared, taboo, forbidden and punishable by infections such as chlamydia, gonorrhoea and HIV, and, in the case of young people, unintended pregnancy. Bhana (2007c) further postulates that parents are unable to talk about sex as pleasure because that would not reconcile with the rhetoric and promotion of childhood innocence. Similarly, parents frequently find it difficult to talk about homosexuality and even masturbation (Mkumbo & Ingham 2010). When discussion about sex does occur they are limited to normative heterosexuality (Kehily 2002). The irony here is that adults indeed do know that children are sexual beings, otherwise why bother with HIV/AIDS education, which is framed around warnings about the dangers of having sex? Clearly, sexual innocence is *not* the experience of many young children, but is wished upon them by parents and other adults.

An interesting paradox presents itself when parental actions expose their children to the manifestations of sex from which they try so hard to shield them. Pupils in the study reported that they had access to pornography through their parents' magazines, tabloids, mobile phones and DVDs. These included pictures of same-sex relationships and various states of nudity and caressing. Two examples are shown in Photos 17 and 18.

Anna (aged 12, School B, South Africa) said she saw a pornographic video when scrolling through her father's phone: 'I deleted them all from my father's phone because it is not right to look at other people's bodies…the woman was jumping from one man to another.' Anna is an example of a girl who shows agency and who is able to make mature decisions on sexuality issues, a fact that most parents may not believe, as they see children as emotionally volatile and susceptible to their bodily urges (Allen 2007). Other children reported finding their parents' pornographic material and watching it. Parents would probably be mortified at the thought of their children having access to their pornographic material. However, repeatedly, the children in our study let us know that they are perceptive, know about sex and are curious about it, even if it means watching pornography. MacKinnon (1984) and Banyard (2010) argue that the danger of pornography is the possible objectification of women whereby boys/men may grow to construct women as objects and treat them as they see them in pornographic films. Furthermore, pornography leads to men constructing who a man is, and how he should behave and treat women according to the pornography they have watched – which is often in dominant and brutal ways. The converse may also be true, with girls/women behaving as they think is 'expected' on the basis of pornography. The theory surrounding the sociology of pornography is quite relevant to our study because in the three countries, pupils talked of watching pornography in local video kiosks or on late night television even if teachers had warned them not to. This, together with the fact that they witness live sex in their neighbourhoods, have easy access to alcohol and drugs, and are open to gift sex, makes them more vulnerable to the negative influences of pornography.

Sexual knowledges from social institutions

Community organisations and social institutions were also mentioned as children's sources of information about sex. These included religious institutions, such as mosques and churches; traditional and cultural agents, such as village elders and traditional healers; non-governmental organisations (NGOs), like USAID in Kenya and loveLife in South Africa; and various health organisations, such as hospitals, clinics and voluntary counselling and testing centres. Pupils in all three countries reported that both Muslim and Christian clerics stressed abstinence for the unmarried, testing before marriage, fidelity for the married and modest dressing. Most pupils, especially in South Africa, blamed the church for only concentrating on 'Jesus stuff' and never talking about sex and relationships. However, they said that in spite of that silence, churchgoers still talked about sex, rape and HIV/AIDS among themselves. Islam's provision that a man can marry many wives was seen as risky. Anna from South Africa asked, 'What if he doesn't know the seventh woman has HIV? He will spread the disease in the house and his children will be HIV-positive.' As will be mentioned below, in Kenya, the overnight Christian prayer meetings (known as *keshas*) were opportunities for young people to have surreptitious sex. Parents who believed in the safety and sanctity of the church allowed their children to attend these *keshas*, little knowing that children took this opportunity to meet their partners and have sex. This is another example of how young people find opportunities for sex despite the protective efforts of adults. It also illustrates the insufficiency of a protective discourse *on its own* and points to the need for more openness with young people.

Practical sexual learning from neighbourhood peers

Living in such an openly sexual world as pupils described, it came as no surprise that some children were also having sex in places like on the street, on buses, at home, at parties, on the beach, in guest houses, in cemeteries and churches, in school and in the bushes (see Photos 19 and 20).

Simiyu, a 15-year-old boy from School A in Kenya, told us that 'after class some pupils do intercourse… in the bush, before they reach home'. And some pupils had sex at home. Jomo, a 12-year-old boy, also from School A in Kenya, said that he not only knew pupils who had had sex at their homes, but also those pupils who fondled each other at school, as will be discussed later. Kantai, a 13-year-old boy from School B, Kenya, had witnessed '[young] people having sexual intercourse at a party…they were completely naked'. Overnight Christian prayer meetings were also an opportunity for young people to engage in sex. Chege, a 13-year-old boy from School B in Kenya, told us that 'at kesha some engage in kissing and others have sex'. In Tanzania pupils said that young people had sex in the bushes and in cemeteries because they could not afford a hotel room and had no other place to do it. These places offered the temporary free and private spaces they needed. There also seemed to be pressure on girls to have sex to keep their boyfriends, as Sakie, a 12-year old girl from School A in South Africa, articulated: 'Some girls often say if they refuse to have [sex] with their boyfriends, the boyfriends will leave them, so they feel compelled to give them.' A reminder of the unequal gender dynamics in sexual relationships and a prime example of how the when, how and where of sex is often controlled by males.

However, it could be argued that since these youths live in such a sexualised world, they overestimate the extent to which their peers are having sex. Apart from those who have seen others having sex, and those who may have had sex themselves, many young people spoke of seeing sexual acts, such as fondling and passionate kissing, and assumed that these acts led to full sex. This is described by

Perkins and Berkowitz (1986) as the social-norms approach. In a study of drinking behaviour, Perkins and Berkowitz (1986) showed that young people frequently overestimate their peers' practice with regard to negative behaviour. This erroneous belief then led to them increasing their own alcohol abuse because of the social norms they believed to be in operation. Correcting this misperceived social norm later curbed their heavy drinking and its related harm. In sexual behaviour, young people also frequently overestimate the proportion of their peers who are sexually active and then attempt to align their own behaviour with these perceived norms (Messer et al. 2011). Messer and colleagues have proposed that these social norms be corrected through social marketing to teens of the real rates of sexual behaviour among teens in an effort to reduce teenage sexual activity.

In-school sources and content of sexual knowledges

Having discussed the everyday, or out-of-school, sexual knowledges that the children in our study possessed, we now present the pupils' formal, or in-school, sources and content of sexual knowledges. We discuss these under four main headings – what was taught; how it was taught; messages from literature and media; and practical learning through observing peers.

What was taught in HIV/AIDS-education lessons: A protective discourse with multiple absences

Teachers played a central role in the quality and quantity of sexual knowledge transmitted to pupils. In most schools, sex and HIV/AIDS education depended on the teacher's disposition towards it. As explained in Chapters 3 and 4, it was only in South Africa that HIV/AIDS education was taught as a stand-alone subject (albeit within the larger learning area, life orientation). In Kenya and Tanzania, teachers had to integrate HIV information into other 'carrier' subjects. In Chapter 4, we described how teachers in Kenya did this in maths and Christian religious education. In Kenya, HIV education was also achieved extramurally through pupils' participation in clubs like the Chill Club, which offered a forum for young people to talk about abstinence informally.

However, in all three countries, pupils reported that they only received a few HIV/AIDS lessons over the course of a school term. South Africa was no exception even if there was the opportunity to teach HIV/AIDS as a component of a dedicated subject, which shows that making space in the timetable for HIV/AIDS education does not guarantee that teachers will teach it. Nonhle (girl, aged 12, School A, South Africa) reported: 'Most of the time we don't have AIDS classes, my teacher does not like giving a lot of AIDS classes.' She added that what she had learnt was mostly from the school library. Therefore, there are other determinants of whether HIV/AIDS education is taught. These is discussed in Chapter 6. Pupils in South Africa blamed teachers for thinking that they were too young to be taught about sex. They said that teachers feared they would experiment with sex if they were taught about it. In a group discussion at School A in South Africa, when asked if they would experiment with sex, children chorused loudly, 'Who wants to experiment with AIDS?' Such a view shows young people's critical thinking and agency. Coleman (2010) writes that in his studies he has found young people to be active agents who can manage the pace of change and select which issues to deal with. It is possible to extrapolate the frustration of these children at receiving little sexual knowledge from teachers. In the discussion, children expressed these frustrations as follows:

Naledi:	The teachers are careful with us because they think we are still young.
Buyelwa:	I think we can be able to process these things in grade 7 or grade 8.
Sisa:	[Last year] they said we were going to learn more in grade 6, but they have not taught us as much.
Pinky:	They think we are too young to know.

Clearly, these children considered themselves old enough to know and reflect Bhana's (2007b: 311) assessment that '[t]hese framings do not encourage young children's active participation in making meaning of HIV, AIDS and sexuality. Nor do they take into account young children's gendered and sexual agency in matters of sexuality rights.'

Sakie, a 12-year-old boy from School A in South Africa, mirrored these frustrations, and spoke of the disadvantages of receiving inadequate HIV/AIDS education: 'We are disadvantaged…we had a project about human rights that asked about private parts, and some of us did not know the words or how to spell them.' He explained that this was because their teacher used euphemisms instead of the correct biological terminology. Foucault (1976: 6) theorises on teachers' protective discourse: 'If sex has been repressed and condemned to prohibition, non-existence, and silence; then the mere fact that one is speaking about it has the appearance of a deliberate transgression. A person who holds forth in such language…upsets established law.' Foucault (1976: 4) also aptly notes, as we recorded at the start of this chapter, that 'everyone knows that "children have no sex", which is why they are forbidden to talk about it, why one closes one's eyes and stops one's ears whenever they show evidence to the contrary'. Both Allen (2007) and Bhana (2007b) argue that the official school culture sees children as asexual and thus strives to regulate their sexuality. This is clearly the case in School A in South Africa. Not only are these children short-changed, but they are not consulted on what should be taught in HIV/AIDS education – a situation that dulls pupils' agency in constructing the HIV/AIDS education that they need and want.[11]

Pupils in all the three countries complained that teachers only taught them facts and did not go deeper by teaching them about issues relating to love and relationships, and the variety of human sexual experience, including ecological aspects, that define sexuality, such as social relationships, emotions and gender issues. This is a finding common in other studies (Allen 2007; Bhana 2007b, 2007c; Campbell & MacPhail 2002; Kiragu 2009). It has been repeatedly shown that, besides a desire to know more than the facts, increasing factual knowledge seldom results in changing behaviour (Bettinghaus 1986). Vygotsky (1978) describes this as trying to separate the cognitive and ecological aspects of learning, which is a false separation because the personal and social aspects of learning are inseparable from the cognitive, a concept that Taylor (2000) terms 'exclusion'.

The pupils in this study reported that the teachers taught facts such as modes of transmission and protection, symptoms, stigma and testing. Children also confirmed that teachers spoke of the ABC mode of protection (Abstain, Be faithful, Condomise), but paid most attention to abstinence, and did not advocate condoms. Chapter 6 provides teachers' perspective and reasoning on this issue. Nevertheless, interviews with pupils revealed that pupils knew a great deal about condoms, though some had misconceptions. For example, in South Africa some pupils said they did not know how to open its wrapping; others in Kenya thought that packs of condoms were small envelopes. Most pupils across the three sites were clear that condoms were used for protection, and in South Africa they even had access to them in clinics and public toilets – although not all pupils from South Africa were aware of this. Pupils in Kenya and South Africa said they knew more about male condoms than female ones ('we don't know where a female condom is fitted…we have not even seen it.'). Busi, a 12-year-old girl from School A, South Africa, talked about how an elder in her community had told her that condoms could break. She said that this was the first time she had learnt this because 'at school we are not told about a condom breaking'. In Kenya and South Africa, pupils reported that there were young people who opted to have sex without a condom, saying that it was more pleasurable that way, or, as Chileza (boy, aged 12, School A, South Africa) argued, 'They do not use a condom because they want to prove they are not infected.' Lear (1997) and Swartz and Bhana (2009) explain that what Chileza said is an issue of trust, namely that insisting on condom use or asking questions about your partner's sexual

11   It can also be argued that teachers are not consulted by policy-makers.

history impacts negatively on the relationship. Pupils in South Africa had knowledge about contraceptives. Buyelwa, (girl, aged 12, School A, South Africa) confidently told us that 'if you want have sex and you are not on injectable contraceptives, you must always use a condom because that condom will prevent sperms from entering you and making you pregnant'.

Condoms were not the only thing lacking in the content of the HIV/AIDS-education curriculum. Zodwa (girl, aged 12, School A, South Africa) gave an example: 'At school they do not test our HIV status, they don't tell us whether you can fall pregnant before you get your periods, they do not even tell us how a girl starts having periods.' This silence on an issue such as pregnancy is dangerous, as pupils in South Africa and Kenya stated that unwanted teenage pregnancies had happened in their schools. For example, within one year in Jomo's school (School A, Kenya), five girls had dropped out because of pregnancy; the boys responsible continued with their education. Nonetheless, Jomo seemed to blame the girls for their predicament, stating that they wanted sex, so they should deal with the consequences. Clearly, the burden of pregnancy falls on the girl and this has been reported as a major reason for poor retention and participation in education among girls (Chege & Sifuna 2006; Elimu Yetu Coalition 2005; Hunt 2009).

Though there were silences and protective discourses from teachers, as evidenced above, in Kenya and South Africa there were some teachers who were open and talked about the exchange of body fluids during sex and the use of condoms. Fahiem (boy, aged 13, School B, South Africa) said that 'teacher teaches that you should always have a condom, you should have safe sex, you should not just sleep with anybody, and to choose the right partner'. Naledi summed it up well:

> There is no need for teachers to be shy because we children already knew about sex. We see it on TV and some of us are already doing it. They must not be ashamed and say we are children. They had the same experience and their teachers were ashamed to speak about these things – but now they must talk to us because AIDS – it is the most infectious disease in South Africa. They must be firm when they talk to us, and they must tell our parents to believe in us as we also believe in them. (Naledi, girl, aged 12, School A, South Africa)

How HIV/AIDS education was taught

In all three countries in our study, we observed that the teaching strategies used in HIV/AIDS education included textbooks, writing on the chalkboard, questions and answers from teachers, examples and experiments to show how the virus spread in the body, storytelling, handouts and worksheets, the internet and role playing. These followed a discernible pattern of teacher *initiates*, student *responds*, teacher gives *feedback* model common in teaching practice. This IRF approach to pedagogy will be discussed in more detail in Chapter 6. Suffice to say that it was perhaps not the most appropriate method for teaching a sensitive subject such as HIV/AIDS. South African pupils described in some detail the learning in their classrooms. Busi (girl, aged 12, School A, South Africa) said: 'Teacher gives us handouts to read. After reading, she asks questions and if we do not put up our hands to answer, she shouts at us.' Sandi (boy, aged 13, School A, South Africa) observed that his teacher preferred the pupils to get their answers from the textbook instead of discussing issues with them. He complained, 'Sometimes if you ask questions, the teacher asks, "Did you not read the story that you were given?"' Teachers assumed that textbook knowledge was adequate, and also used the textbook to mask their own discomfort and lack of confidence in teaching these topics. Busi related how some teachers opted to walk out of class rather than answer an 'embarrassing' question:

> We were doing group work and wanted to know whether a man who sleeps with another man can get infected with HIV or fall pregnant. Ms Yeki did not answer us, she walked out of the class… promising she would tell us at a later stage. (Busi, girl, aged 12, School A, South Africa)

This teacher's response could be a combination of the protective and childhood innocence discourses that works to divorce HIV and AIDS from sexuality (Bhana 2007c), while also masking her discomfort at talking about sex and same-sex relationships with pupils (Kehily 2002). It may also be the result of inherent traditional authoritarianism, whereby adults often reserve the rights to knowledge (Jewkes et al. 2005, Tabulawa 1997). And indeed, it may also reflect a situation in which the teacher is expected to teach more than she knows, has experienced, or believes in. A situation which is both personal and difficult is worsened if the teacher is unprepared or unwilling to take charge and break the silence – or, in this case, cross the normative boundaries of heterosexuality. As Burbules and Hansen (1997) suggest, a teacher contends with social values that are in tension with one another, and can hardly serve the interests of all pupils. However, because the teacher's job is to teach, other adults expect them to talk about sex, even if they are neither confident nor comfortable to do so.

Another teaching strategy apparent in South Africa was demonstrated when a teacher used one of the pupils as an example to illustrate a point – with unintended consequences. A boy explained:

> Sometimes when teachers talk about sex and say we mustn't do it because it is dangerous, she would mention a learner's name in class, others would laugh, so the learner would get embarrassed as others think she does sex, although a teacher may be just making an example. (Xolani, boy, aged 12, School A, South Africa)

Xolani further explained that learners were not happy to be used in these types of examples that displayed them as sexually active. This example, which seemed to create stigma in South Africa, exemplifies the teachers' challenge of being sensitive to all pupils in a world of contested social mores. For this age group, children do not want to appear to adults and to others as being sexually active, as this is publicly viewed as wrong. Bhana (2007b: 319) explains that these contradictions show children '… very clearly struggling to present themselves as the ideal child and to project innocence. They adopt the positionings that adults have set for them.'

Pupils also suggested ways to improve learning, such as single-sex lessons where they would feel more comfortable to ask personal questions without the opposite sex present; watching films that portray the 'shocking truth' about HIV/AIDS; and having exams on the subjects to compel them to learn the information. However, Vuai, a 13-year-old boy from Tanzania, said that girls were given more information on sex and HIV/AIDS than boys, and implored teachers to talk to boys as well. There were some pupils who felt that the teachers were more effective than their parents at talking to them about sex and AIDS. In a classroom observation in South Africa, Lonwabo explained why this might be the case:

> It's because a teacher illustrates on everything as compared to a parent who may be shy. But when you are educated by the teacher, students get a chance to ask questions concerning that issue… with parents you get less time for discussion…maybe s/he gets home at 9 p.m. (Lonwabo, boy, School A, South Africa)

Despite other criticisms children may have, this statement captures the important role of the teacher in offering children HIV/AIDS education.

Other in-school sources: Literature and the media

Various forms of literature and media were also common sources of sexual knowledges in the school, such as books, newspapers, magazines, posters, wall paintings, banners, graffiti, messages on clothes, chalkboards, drama and role plays, and the internet (in South Africa only). Photos 21 and 22 show some of these sources captured by children during their photovoice projects.

Practical sexual learning from peers: Pupils' sexual worlds in school

Not surprisingly, peers were also an active source of information for children, either verbally or through observation and practice. Photos 23 and 24 illustrate pupils in Tanzania teaching each other both formally and informally.

Away from the HIV/AIDS education in the classrooms, pupils' interviews revealed an active and sophisticated sexual world within the school – a world which (from the discussion above) did not seem to be discussed or engaged with by teachers during classroom learning. In all three countries, pupils spoke openly about the sexual urges that they were experiencing as maturing teenagers. Boys in Kenya described their female companions as 'hyper' and talking loudly and too much; they interpreted this as a result of the excitement that came with puberty, as Mbaya and Shitandi comment:

> Now that their breasts are out and they just talk too much…they don't listen…they like shaking their hips in class…they are looking for boyfriends. (Mbaya, boy, aged 13, School A, Kenya)

> When a girl is an adolescent she is never calm, she is all over the place shaking/swaying [her hips] in front of us boys. They must show off…she is doing it so that her boyfriend can see…and her boyfriend will boast to us 'that one is mine'…and when he says that some of us envy him, while others will tell him that it is too early to have a relationship. (Shitandi, boy, aged 12, School A, Kenya)

Boys in the same school also reported that the girls intentionally aroused them, although they did admit they were not sure whether it was out of playful curiosity or serious intent:

> They touch each other's breasts in front of us…they even tap you to get your attention so that you can see them do it…it makes us get that strong feeling of wanting them. (Simiyu, boy, aged 15, School A, Kenya)

Jomo, a 12-year-old boy from the same school, confided that pupils often went behind the school buildings to fondle each other. One of his peers, Irungu, reported that having multiple partners either for sex or petting was common:

> There is a boy in class eight…he is 17…he has four girlfriends…one is in class six, two in class seven, and the other in class five…the girls know each other, but they don't know they are dating one boy. (Irungu, boy, aged 14, School A, Kenya)

He further explained that such an arrangement was accepted as long as the girls involved were friends. There were similar examples of multiple partners in their neighbourhoods at home. Pointing to one of his photographs that showed a boy with two girls near his home, Shitandi explained:

> These two girls both like this boy…we see them all the time in the streets…When this one meets him they make love and when this other one meets him they make love…They don't mind as long as you are sharing with your friend. (Shitandi, boy, aged 12, School A, Kenya)

The examples given by these Kenyan boys show how adolescents, especially young men, are experiencing sexual urges and exploring how to deal with them. However, it is true that some of these pupils are somewhat older than the average age for primary school, and are in an isolated rural area with very few recreational facilities, which may contribute to their behaviour, and such behaviour might differ from that of younger pupils. Although our data did not capture young women talking as explicitly as these young men, nevertheless young women were not silent on issues of the dynamics of love, desire and seduction in the schools. Girls refer to the multiple partners that boys have, and the many ways in which they actively pursue sexual relationships within the school context. Rifquah, from South Africa, made the following observation about sex and relationships, which shows a sophisticated understanding of sexual dynamics, and portrays insight, knowledge and a lack of innocence:

> I thought about it. Some people have sex because they are alone, some people have sex because they love each other, some people have sex because they are paid to have sex. (Rifquah, girl, aged 12, School B, South Africa)

On a number of occasions, especially in Cape Town and Mombasa, researchers observed overt sexual behaviour among pupils. These observations included a 12-year-old boy staring at the behind of a girl who had walked past; two pupils locked in a romantic embrace in a classroom during an afternoon sports event; and a boy playing with and showing other boys (and the next day, a girl) his aroused penis, at which they laughed.

This sexual knowledge and these actions evident among these children stand in contrast to the protective and innocent discourses from parents and teachers. A paradox presents itself. Adults attempt to repress sexuality (especially children's sexuality) and police, monitor and regulate the production of (hetero)-sexual identities (Allen 2007; Kehily 2002). However, this repression, in turn, produces resistance and a multiplicity of sexual discourses that are the very opposite of those intended by adults (Foucault 1976; Kehily 2002). As Kehily (2002: 59) says, 'acts of prohibition and censorship produce and enlarge the very things they seek to deny'. The data we present here provides a good example of resisting the sexual repression/protective discourse that the adults have put in place. Far from adhering to it, the pupils display sophisticated and knowledgeable sexual lives. Much of their behaviour (especially among those who are older and still in primary school) predisposes them to HIV and other sexually transmitted infections, and early parenting. Because sexuality within the school prevails in such a powerful way, scholars such as Kehily (2002) have constructed it as a framework in itself. She distinguishes between the official school curriculum/pedagogy and student cultures. It is these student cultures at school that encapsulate children's sexual worlds in the school.

How contexts affect sexual knowledges – A comparison

In this chapter we have presented data that illustrate children's two primary worlds – school and out of school (i.e. their homes and communities). Table 5.1 summarises in broad brush strokes how these knowledges contrast and differ. However, as we have already alluded, these worlds are not separate in reality. Children bring their knowledge from home and community into the school, although they frequently leave it at the door of the classroom. The secret sexual lives they live in the corridors, behind the toilets and through talking to their friends are seldom discussed in the classroom.

TABLE 5.1 *Comparison of sources and contents of children's sexual knowledges in and out of school*

Out of school

Source of sexual knowledge	Its content
• Home (parents and relatives). • Neighbourhood (open spaces, such as streets, bushes, school, buses, beach). • Recreational spaces (beer dens, parties, discos, brothels, guest houses). • People (peers, gang members, older sexual partners, such as sugar mommies and daddies, and village elders). • Media (videos, films, mobile phones, TV, pornography, newspapers, magazines, banners, posters). • Social institutions (NGOs, churches and keshas, mosques, cemeteries). • Health organisations (hospitals, clinics, voluntary counselling centres, local administration/council centres).	• Observing adults and peers having sex in public places. Sometimes observing group sex, or same-sex activities. Seeing members of a gang masturbating. • Pupils' and others' use of substances such as illicit brew, bhang and dagga – and how people behave sexually when 'high' or 'drunk'. • Hearing and speaking 'dirty' language that pupils would perhaps not normally speak at school. • Having sex and relationships for money or 'gifts'. • Sexual assault by peers and relatives (incest and paedophilia). Special danger from male youths who are drug addicts and have dropped out of school. • Accessing pornography from parents and video shows in kiosks on late night television. • Abstinence message from parents, church and mosques.

In school

Source of sexual knowledge	Its content
• People (peers and teachers). • Activities (lessons, clubs, drama, role play). • Media (textbooks, posters, wall paintings, chalkboard, library, internet, messages on clothes, billboards, graffiti).	• Facts about HIV/AIDS – definitions, symptoms, transmission, prevention, testing and stigma. • Facts about transmission – through breast milk, a cut or wound, deep kissing, mother to child, a razor, sex, a syringe or injection and sharing a toothbrush. • Protection – abstinence, being faithful to one partner, and condoms (generally not advocated). • Contraceptives (especially injectable types) from peers. • Abstinence and avoidance of sex with sugar daddies/mommies; avoiding prostitution. • Warnings about the consequences of unwanted pregnancy and drug abuse. • Euphemisms used for sex and sexual organs – with only a few teachers being 'open' or 'free'.

Now that we have understood the sources and content of the pupils' sexual knowledges, the next question is how their contexts and experiences influence the acquisition of sexual knowledges. As evidenced above, their home environments have exposed them to 'live sex' because social control, rules and regulations are limited in poor communities where privacy, sobriety, safety and adequate resources are in short supply. Such an environment often rids the child of 'the innocence of childhood' along with a structured and organised way of learning because sexual exposure is explicit and unconstrained. As a result, children living in these environments are highly sexually aware. Good examples are the children in Photos 12 and 13. Both children will grow up in an environment where they see people taking drugs and having sexual intercourse in the open. Sex on display occurs perhaps because houses are small and recreational spaces and opportunities for privacy limited. So people necessarily inhabit open spaces for their personal space and freedom – including their sexual lives. These public sexual lives that children see and from which they derive everyday knowledge are in sharp contrast to the formal curriculum in school. The insulation and boundary between the two is strongly defined and clear. The school context offers factual information and a protective discourse removed from the pupils' lived experiences, where everyday knowledges provide unfiltered information that children could benefit from discussing. As Kehily (2002: 67) summarises:

> The official classroom task sees sex education in terms of technical knowledge, details of biology and sexual health to be learned and accumulated, while pupil interactions [their everyday sexual worlds] stress the importance of the experiential and the instrumental role of the peer group in key aspects of social learning.

Our data show that children have a knowledgeable and sophisticated sexual world both in and out of the school – and one that they are fully capable of articulating. A protective and repressive discourse does not seem appropriate for these young people. They know about sexual encounters and see it in buses, bushes, brothels, cemeteries and *keshas*. Some are engaged in sexual activity themselves. Their voices captured in our study show that they would want teachers (and other adults) to engage with these experiences in a comprehensive and interactive way. Arguably, pupils trust their teachers and want to be able to confide in them. How do teachers respond to these implicit and overt requests for change to the way things have always been done? This is the topic of Chapter 6, in which we consider pupils', teachers' and other stakeholders' perceptions of and dilemmas about HIV/AIDS education.

CHAPTER 6

AIDS education in the classroom: Perceptions and dilemmas

In Chapters 2, 4 and 5 we described in some detail the social and sexual contexts of the lives of the children in our study. We have shown through these context descriptions and through the photovoice exercise that in all the schools in our study, pupils reported a defined boundary between their everyday, or horizontal, sexual knowledges (mainly out of school) and their formal, in-school, or vertical, sexual knowledges. In this chapter we present perceptions about current HIV and sex education from the three main actors in schooling – pupils, teachers and community stakeholders (including parents). To understand pupils' perceptions of their current AIDS-education lessons, we asked them to plan, perform and video-record a two- to three-minute mini-documentary depicting what they currently learnt (content) and how (pedagogy). The videos were recorded using the cameras we had given them for the photovoice activity. The second part of their task was to create another documentary in which they role played how they would like these lessons to be. Therefore, in total, pupils planned, acted and recorded two role plays, the first showing their current HIV/AIDS-education lessons; the second showing how they desired their HIV/AIDS-education lessons to be. In all eight schools a total of 21 role plays were performed and recorded, as described in Chapter 2.

Once completed, we showed a group of teachers in each school the second video (how the pupils desired their HIV/AIDS lessons to be). After watching the video, teachers and researchers engaged in a discussion about what they had just watched. We also interviewed these teachers individually about their experiences with HIV/AIDS education in their teaching careers. We also recruited a group of parents and community stakeholders in each school in order to obtain their opinion on HIV/AIDS education in the school. As a result, this chapter presents the voices of the three main actors in the school community on the subject of HIV/AIDS and sex education – pupils, teachers, and community members. It concludes with a reflection on the nature and interplay of social space for each constituency.

Pupils' role plays

Various themes emerged in the pupils' role plays. The theme of the first role play was similar in all three countries, where children's role plays showed that their current HIV/AIDS education was mainly teacher-driven, as discussed later. For the second role play, themes varied in the different countries. For example, South African pupils' documentaries focused on what they wanted to know, such as the biology of HIV/AIDS, its progression through the body and how to use a condom. In Tanzania pupils showed that they sought participatory ways of learning using group work, role plays and media. In Kenya the pupils portrayed various moral stories about HIV/AIDS. These included that of a young woman exchanging sex for a job, only to contract HIV/AIDS from her boss; the shock and denial that came with the realisation that one was infected; a mother trying to influence her daughter to stop schooling and join her in prostitution; and pupils sneaking out of class to have sex. These role plays were rich, student-driven from start to finish and enabled our pupils to voice their views (no matter how sensitive or incriminating) in a depersonalised way.

Children's perceptions of their current HIV/AIDS-education lessons

As highlighted by a number of findings in Hardman et al. (2008) in Nigeria; Tabulawa (1997) in Malawi; Altinyelken (2010) in Uganda; and Dembélé and Lefoka (2007) in various contexts in sub-Saharan Africa, classroom pedagogy in developing countries has been dominated by teacher-directed, rote-learning methods. In these classrooms, it has been noted that pupils are often not involved in the teaching and learning process, and instead become passive recipients of knowledge. Teacher talk dominates lessons and pupils only occasionally participate by being asked to respond to factual answers based on recall of information from a textbook or what the teacher has just said. Such teacher-directed classes are likely to restrict the development of children's thinking and creative problem solving (Freire 1970). Through the pupils' videos, we captured similar findings in the three countries in this study to support this conclusion.

Teacher-driven talk and choral answers

Role plays by pupils in Tanzania and Kenya echoed what Hardman et al. (2008) found in Nigeria: that teachers expected pupils to repeat in chorus what was written on the board. In one instance in School B in Tanzania, the teacher began the question with the statement 'What did I say the causes of HIV/AIDS are?' and the pupils shouted back the answer in chorus. In role plays from the same school pupils showed how teachers asked pupils to name sharp objects that could transmit the HIV virus from infected blood. However, the teacher did not let the pupils volunteer the answers; instead, he read them out aloud from the textbook, with pupils repeating after him in chorus.

Teaching through the use of closed and leading questioning was another prevalent practice displayed in pupils' documentaries. The pupils in Kenya and Tanzania acted out teachers asking them questions like, 'What did I say about nails and sharp objects? Can they cause AIDS?' To which the pupils chorused back 'yes'. After the chorused answer, there was no follow-up from the teacher other than asking another closed and leading question, and this went on throughout the role play. Such a mode of answering results in pupils merely following each other's answers and allows no time to listen to, reflect on or analyse each other's views. It also means teachers uncritically accept the group's response and does not allow them to hear individual responses and so follow up on pupils' individual learning, growth and discernment. Voices of introverted children or those with special needs may also be drowned out in these chorused answers, so they are particularly disadvantaged by such teaching methods. Hardman et al. (2008) argue that chorus answers not only restrict individual pupils' cognitive and linguistic development, but can also instil a culture of 'indifferent attention' in what is being discussed in the class. It can encourage pupils to block out classroom deliberation and allow their thoughts to wander. Furthermore, a child is more likely to develop 'restricted' or 'public code' responses, as he or she is learning in a classroom environment where mostly only monosyllabic sentences and responses are expected (Bernstein 1990a). There are several factors that may lead teachers to teach this way. Some have low levels of teacher education with restricted pedagogical methods at their disposal. They are frequently confronted with large class sizes, and limited space or resources for interactive teaching, and little opportunity for providing individual attention to pupils (Altinyelken 2010; Dembélé and Lefoka 2007). Pedagogy is also dependent on teachers' epistemologies and their views on the purpose of education. For example, their view of education may be that teachers *transmit* knowledge to pupils (Altinyelken 2010; Tabulawa 1997), and so their practice merely follows this view.

Being rebuffed by teachers

Pupils showed that asking questions could result in punishment and harsh responses from their teachers. For example, when one pupil from School A in Tanzania asked, 'What if someone is pricked with a rusted nail, and we do not know who was hurt by that nail before, can he get HIV?' the teacher answered, 'I do not have time for stupid questions!' With such a rebuff, the knowledge sought by the pupil is not acquired and the opportunity to develop pupils' critical thinking skills is lost. Such a situation also exacerbates the gap or hierarchy between teachers and pupils, and eventually the pupils may be discouraged from exploring knowledge by asking questions. Teachers may choose this route of rebuffing questions because of the time pressures of a busy curriculum and large classes, an inability to answer or they embrace the protective discourse – the discourse of childhood innocence – to which we have previously referred. Often teachers are expected to teach more than they know, have been trained for, have experienced, or believe in (Allen 2007; Bhana 2007a, 2007b, 2007c; Burbules & Hansen 1997). Instead of enduring the embarrassment of looking ignorant in front of pupils, teachers compensate for this lack of knowledge or uneasiness by being harsh and authoritative. Perhaps this behaviour also results from the authoritarianism and respect for elders that is inherent and prevalent in many African societies. The authority of age is still widely respected, as it is associated with wisdom (Jewkes et al. 2005; Tabulawa 1997). Tabulawa (1997: 195) links this tradition to practice in the modern-day classroom, terming the traditional notion of authority as 'cultural baggage':

> Because these structures of domination and subordination have been internalised, students and teachers carry them to the classroom as their cultural baggage, which in turn informs their actions and respective classroom roles…the authoritarian pedagogical style mediates the classroom and the wider social structure, that is, it is through the pedagogical style that the wider social structure finds expression in the classroom.

Lack of answers or feedback from teachers

Similar findings by Dembélé and Lefoka (2007) in Lesotho, and Hardman et al. (2008) in Nigeria report that teachers initiated a question and expected a certain response, but did not follow up on the response given by the pupils or provide feedback. Sinclair and Coulthard (1992) call this 'teacher-pupil talk', or the initiation-response-follow-up (IRF) approach we alluded to in Chapter 4. The teacher initiates the conversation and learning, the pupil responds and the teacher gives feedback. The IRF model could have been used by teachers to institute interactions in the classroom (White 2003; Yu 2009). However, to a greater extent in our schools, the pupils' role plays suggested that the IRF model rarely reached the level of response from them let alone the follow-up. For example, pupils at School B in Tanzania role played their teacher asking factual questions in the form of an incomplete sentence and then answering the question herself or after a pause expecting a chorus response. Not surprisingly, pupils in that school showed in role play that they did not bother asking questions and were unwilling to answer questions that were posed. There was also no attempt by the teacher to rephrase unanswered questions, or follow up as to why pupils did not answer. Instead the teacher herself, after receiving no response from pupils, went ahead and gave answers to the question from the textbook. Similarly, in South Africa, pupils described their teachers as standing in front of the classroom defining HIV/AIDS and asking the pupils to repeat the definition. For example, Fahiem, a 13-year-old boy from School B in South Africa, said: 'My teacher stands in front of the class and writes on the board what HIV stands for…then we repeat.' Such practice is bound to deprive pupils of the opportunity to think of a possible answer.

In fact, Hardman et al. (2008: 58) observed that pupils can tell from the intonation that the teacher expects them to finish the sentence, what he refers to as a 'cued elicitation'. The teacher in such instances actually sends the message of being all-knowing, the 'banker of knowledge', and the pupils are 'containers' or 'receptacles' waiting to be 'filled' by the teacher (Freire 1970). In such a banking model, the pupils record, memorise and repeat phrases without understanding what they really mean, or without realising the true significance of the knowledge. It is possible that this banking model is culturally driven and facilitated by the 'structures of domination and subordination' described by Tabulawa (1997). Freire (1970) writes that it is a model that develops passivity instead of the life skills of critical thinking, decision-making and confidence to voice one's opinion and deal with one's emotions.

Children's expression of their pedagogical preferences

In the preceding section, we highlighted the current ways in which HIV/AIDS education is carried out in the classrooms, as reflected in pupils' first documentaries. In this section we discuss the second role play, which mainly portrayed pupils' desire for interactive pedagogy in HIV/AIDS and sex education. The need to include interactive pedagogy in the classrooms of sub-Saharan primary schools cannot be emphasised enough. Pupils in all three countries in which we conducted research want the same elements to be present in HIV- and sex-education classes. They want to know more about the pandemic, but in an environment that allows them to take ownership and be confident to participate in the process of constructing knowledge. They are '"more robust, articulate and willing to be heard" than adults had assumed' (Craig 2003, as cited in Bragg 2007: 14). For example, in South Africa, Naledi, a 13-year-old girl from School A, wanted to know 'what happens when a condom breaks', but said that her teacher would not answer that. The example of Busi from South Africa, who wanted to know more about infection among gay men, as mentioned in Chapter 5, also fits in here. Her plea was for teachers not to walk out of the classroom when asked a difficult question, but to face pupils openly and answer their queries.

Moral stories

In the case of Kenya, pupils' second role plays (i.e. the method of sex and AIDS education that they desired) were mainly moral stories reflecting the realities of pupils' lives and the topics they wished to discuss. These included the exchange of sex for money, jobs or gifts, such as mobile phones, cars and going abroad. They discussed how these realities affected their domestic lives. Pupils in Kenya also revealed the need for coping skills and strategies in personal HIV/AIDS management. For example, one of the role plays showed people not knowing what to do when they found out they were infected with HIV. Their role plays also revealed the social pressures to have sex. A role play from School B showed how a poor and sick mother implored her daughter to look for a job to support the family materially. When she looked for a job, the boss wanted to have sex with her first. Because she was desperate for the job, she had sex with him oblivious of the fact that he was HIV-positive. The play ends with the boss dying and the girl and her mother distraught because she too is infected. A role play from School C was about a girl whose mother was a prostitute and could not afford her school fees. The mother tried to persuade the girl to join her in prostitution, but she refused saying she wanted to complete her education and become successful.

Such role plays depict the convoluted dilemmas children face in their lives outside of school and can be good entry points for dialogue on pupils' lives. Role plays as entry points to dialogue can 'depersonalise' such sensitive issues. They give the pupils the opportunity to highlight the structural drivers that either contribute to increased individual risk of exposure to HIV or compromise children's ability to protect themselves from infection (Campbell 2003; Gupta et al. 2008). These stories challenge assumptions that once people acquire factual information (as the pupils did from their teachers – at least to some extent, although their deeper questions were frequently ignored), they are able to make rational decisions that change their risky sexual behaviour (Campbell 2003). The stories demonstrate that people do not always have the power to make individual safe choices, and that there are stronger social, structural, and cultural forces that shape people's sexual worlds – including those of children.

Participatory learning

Pupils in School C in Tanzania expressed a strong desire to discuss sexuality issues in small groups. In one of their documentaries they displayed a sophisticated understanding of how this group work might look. They first acted out a role play on drug abuse and its impact on the spread of HIV/AIDS with the 'class' watching (this was a role play within a role play). The 'teacher' then divided the class into groups for discussion. The discussion was guided by questions such as how can we educate the community on the danger of HIV/AIDS? What kinds of thing should be taught in schools to prevent such behaviour (drug abuse)? And how can we share the knowledge we have with those who are engaged in undesirable behaviour? The pupil playing the role of the teacher facilitated the group work by reiterating the questions, providing support to the groups by answering their questions and clarifying their queries about the task at hand. He provided multiple opportunities for group members to share their views by asking if anyone had a different answer.

At School B in Tanzania, pupils role played watching a film on television about teenage life and then held group discussions on how the teenager portrayed in the 'film' could cope with life and what the community could do to guide adolescents. The 'teacher' in the role play allowed each group to critique the response of the other in a manner that resulted in engaged discussions among students. Points made were summarised, challenged and clarified. The pedagogy displayed in the pupils' second video reflects a 'weakly framed' curriculum, where both pupils and teachers are able to influence content and pedagogy (Bernstein 1971). These documentaries, especially from Tanzania, expressed a strong desire for new platforms and pedagogical methods for discussing HIV/AIDS. Children spoke of how group discussions between learners and teachers could create space to hear each other's realities and come up with workable solutions to difficult dilemmas.

Open and in-depth explanations

Clearly, children sought discourses of contextual understanding, including understanding their own sexual lives, and their lived realities of dealing with friends and family members facing life with HIV infection, sexual temptations and exposure. This is in contrast to the predominant discourse of protection they currently experience in their school contexts. Pupils in South Africa were specific about the in-depth knowledge they sought. They wanted their teachers to show practical examples of how HIV/AIDS spread from one person to another, how to put on a condom, how an unborn child got infected with HIV, the origin of the virus, why it is incurable and why people who used condoms still got infected. They also wanted to understand the pandemic from the perspective of those who are dealing with it, and were keen for opportunities for activism. For instance, Naledi from South Africa said, 'I would like to see people who have AIDS…they could tell us about AIDS.' They were also keen to make posters and hold candle-light vigils for those who had died of AIDS in order to make the community aware of the epidemic. These requests for in-depth knowledge, changed pedagogy and the interrogation of moral tales as lived realities all stress children's need for AIDS and sex education that deals with everyday occurrences in their lives. These children want more relevant, deeper HIV and sex education in contrast to their current experience of being containers for the transmission of selected factual information, of which most are already aware.

The power of pupil consultation

This section has presented the classroom reality of HIV/AIDS education through the pupils' lens. In all three countries, it is a pedagogy that is predominantly teacher initiated, with pupils giving chorus answers. It has also depicted the form of HIV/AIDS education that children desired to have, namely one that consults them and is participatory, with open and in-depth information. The process and activities that we undertook in this study helped highlight that when consulted (e.g. through photography, interviews and role plays), pupils have a huge contribution to make and rather than passive objects, they can be active players in the education system (Rudduck 2005). Consultation gives them the space to create and share knowledge.

Teachers' perceptions of their HIV/AIDS education practice

Having presented pupils' current and desired experience of HIV/AIDS education, this section now explores their teachers' views on sex and AIDS education. We asked teachers to evaluate their current teaching practice, their responses to pupils' suggestions on the HIV/AIDS education they want (based on pupils' video documentaries), and, lastly, we engaged teachers in a discussion on the social space in which HIV/AIDS education is conducted. As described in Chapter 2, four to six teachers per school were interviewed individually and later engaged as a group (in a focus group discussion, or FGD) to discuss children's 'desired' documentaries. This section draws on both of these sets of data.

Teachers' analysis of their current practice

Through the interviews and FGDs, we were able to tease out teachers' judgements of their current practice in HIV/AIDS education. Three main themes emerged: the content of lessons, pedagogy and self-evaluations of effectiveness.

Content – mainly factual

As described by children in Chapter 5, teachers confirmed that they mainly taught the facts of transmission and prevention, and relied on the textbook for this information. Ms Nafula from School A, Kenya, added, 'We don't talk about sex.' The main fear from teachers was that if they did, the pupils would experiment. 'If you just talk [about] all the areas concerning sex…they might go and practise it,' Ms Nafula argued. This belief leads to teachers being careful, weighing their words and being silent on sexual issues. The experiences of these teachers are similar to observations from Bhana's (2007a, 2007b, 2007c) study in South Africa, where teachers felt comfortable talking about HIV/AIDS as a medical issue, but were silent on sex as a mode of transmission. Teachers from School B, South Africa, were emphatic. Ms Van Zyl said that the message she gave was, 'No to condom use…abstaining…and that they must stick to one partner.' Ms Carpenter said that in spite of teachers dissuading children from using condoms, 'some naughty ones' still brought them to school, blew them up like balloons and played with them. Some teachers were more flexible and taught pupils to 'wait till the right time'. Ms Carpenter spelled out her message:

> I tell them to wait until they are older and mentally ready to think of having sex…I tell my class that it is in our nature to have sex, to think about it, and have our brains active on it but I tell them to think responsibly.

Some teachers taught about sexual abuse because they were aware of the extent to which it occurred in pupils' communities, as reported by children in Chapter 5, though, as Ms Richards explained, they did not give details. Ms Papier talked about how she taught children not to allow anybody to touch them, and what to do if someone did. She said that in her class, more common than questions about sex were questions about sexual abuse: 'It is not about sex as such but more about "teacher, what must I do when somebody touches me?" and I don't think they understand what is a good and a bad touch.' So although the teachers from School B in South Africa articulated the point best, almost all the teachers who participated in FGDs spoke of their focus as being factual and avoided the subject of sex or condoms unless they were talking about protecting children against abuse.

Pedagogy

With regard to pedagogy, in all three countries, the activities that teachers reported they used in class were role plays, oral and written stories, discussions, question and answer, basic information about the body and the transmission of the disease from textbooks or other media, singing and acting about HIV/AIDS, reading handouts, maths and statistics to discuss rates in a particular place, providing real-life examples and activist involvement in World AIDS Day activities. These matched those mentioned by the pupils in Chapter 5. In Tanzania Mr Manage from School C said that they borrowed from popular TV adverts and based lessons on these. He gave an example of an advert where a girl rejected a sexual advance from a shopkeeper by responding *sidanganyiki* (Swahili for 'I cannot be deceived'). He said that teachers in his school often repeated the same slogan to their students, saying that 'if anyone approaches them…they should tell them *sidanganyiki*'. This is a good example of how the media can have a positive influence in teaching practice. These methods appear to be quite comprehensive. Pupils do acknowledge a variety of methods, but hint at the extent to which one or two are favoured.

How teachers judged their effectiveness

When asked to evaluate their effectiveness in teaching AIDS- and sex-education classes, teachers employed different strategies to do so. They thought they had taught well when children either asked or could answer lots of questions, or when the stories they told seemed relevant and/or resonated well with pupils' own lives. They also knew that they were more effective if they used stories and role plays. Teachers from School C in Kenya also eavesdropped on pupils during break time to hear what they were talking about, and checked on its accuracy, as related by Mr Matu: 'If you pass near them you might hear what they are talking about…sometimes they are usually right, but sometimes their facts are jumbled up. I think they are exposed to so many things around them, both immoral and good, it confuses them.' However, although teachers were keen to show how their teaching resulted in accurate fact retention, we have already shown how the literature argues that acquisition of knowledge, though necessary, is not in itself sufficient or a guarantee of behaviour change (Aggleton & Campbell 2000; Campbell 2003). As presented in Chapter 5, there are other determinants of behaviour, perhaps even more influential than knowledge. Ms Dube from School A, South Africa, summarises the circulation of knowledge and its contextual effects:

> It is hard to affirm that you have done something effective with these children because…when they go back to their communities…they meet with those who…are streetwise…and are easily influenced…and they forget all that you have taught them. Yes, there are those few who would remember what I taught and stick to it but some would care less…and say, 'I am on my own, I can do this, the teacher won't see me.'

However, there were instances when even if the pupils proved that they had understood what was taught, their selective responses caused further problems – in one case perpetuating stigma. In Tanzania, Ms Aisha (School A) narrated that she knew her teaching had been effective when a child hurt himself and was bleeding and other children were scared to help, as they did not want to risk coming into contact with blood. In the same school, a girl reported to the teacher that she had refused to eat at home because when cooking, her mother had put the ladle in her mouth and thus 'contaminated the food'. These fear responses from children might be normal for their developmental stage, or fear might have been instilled in them through the ways in which teachers chose to teach. Perhaps teachers failed to explain in detail, or did not check pupils' understanding by asking questions, listening and interpreting answers, and then building on these understandings. Examples include explaining about using gloves and how saliva is not dangerous unless imbibed in copious amounts.

Teachers' responses to pupils' suggestions on the kind of HIV/AIDS education they want

Reflecting on their practice during initial interviews produced little self-criticism in the teachers. However, when teachers watched the pupils' video documentaries their responses were profound. These simple videos seemed to open the teachers' minds and paved the way for reflection on practice (Freire 1970).

Positive learning

Mr Moi from School B, Kenya, commented:

> They are suggesting different methods of teaching, like discussion and drama. And in drama they take part fully, meaning if teachers also started teaching using drama, they would be very effective where learning is concerned.

Ms Van Zyl (School B, South Africa) felt that the pupils were more active in the videos than they were in her class and accepted these videos as displaying helpful guiding principles: 'I am just surprised at certain children speaking and enjoying the class when they don't usually speak in my class. So how they are teaching is also giving us ideas'.

Both of these quotations demonstrate that the video documentaries produced by children stimulated learning and reflection among the teachers. Ms Ndura from Kenya reflected on the videos she had seen and saw drama as a way in which pupils 'practised' what they were taught. Several videos in Kenya showed that there was conflict between parents and teachers, with the parents physically attacking a teacher in one video from School A. Teachers from this school said that there was sometimes violence at school between teachers and parents. When asked how parents and teachers could amicably work together, Mr Ndegwa suggested that dialogue should happen in ordinary parent-teacher meetings: 'Parents and teachers can sit together *and teachers can sensitise them*…on the responsibility he or she has on the child.' Mr Ndegwa reflects the understanding that it is their job to tell parents what is best for their children, and illustrates the power dynamics present between teachers and parents – a topic to which we will later return.

Some videos in Tanzania and South Africa showed pupils learning from watching HIV/AIDS documentaries. Teachers applauded this because they perceived it as a way for pupils to better comprehend by seeing reality. Similarly, Mr Manage from School C in Tanzania said that field trips to visit people living with HIV/AIDS would be effective, but the problem was that the school could not afford to hire a bus for such trips. 'They will never forget the patient they see with their own eyes. This will make real what we teach in class,' he said. Another suggestion from Ms Kafuma (School B, Tanzania) was for the government to provide them with HIV/AIDS textbooks for all classes, including lower primary. She felt that this would promote self-study, and teachers and parents would have a common source to which to refer, hence minimising contradictory messages. However, Ms Nkasawe, Ms Dube and Mr Zulu (School A, South Africa) said that some of their pupils (and the pupils' parents) could not read properly or were 'lazy to read', and, therefore, such a strategy would have its challenges. Teachers also agreed that the sophisticated sexual knowledges that pupils displayed in the videos were real, as they were exposed to these issues in their communities. Mr Zulu added that even if children knew about other modes of transmission, they displayed 'curiosity about how one got infection through the sperm and vagina'.

Teachers' growing self-reflection

Not all comments made by teachers were positive. We specifically avoided showing teachers children's 'current' documentaries, since we thought these might offend teachers, and we had expected that children might exaggerate the nature of their current sex- and AIDS-education classes. To some extent, we were right – children frequently highlighted what they found 'boring' and what they immediately remembered rather than providing comprehensive portrayals of their current realities. However, when teachers watched the 'desired' videos, they also reacted to some of the negative portrayals of teachers in these documentaries. For example, in a moral tale from Kenya, Mr Oile (School A) was not happy that in one video the teacher had forgotten to bring the chalk with him, and, therefore, had to leave the classroom for a few minutes, during which time two students sneaked out of class to have sex in the bushes. Neither did he like it that the teacher had to excuse himself to the students before he went to get the chalk. He said: 'To me the teacher was not prepared…his coming without chalk resulted to the pupils having a chance to sneak out. Otherwise if he was fully prepared with all the learning aids in the class that would not have happened.'

The story went on to show the pupils being caught having sex in the bush and the teacher sending them home to get their parents. Mr Owino complained about the lack of confidentiality that ensued:

> The mistake the teacher did was that he solved this case in front of the class so everyone heard what the two pupils had done. He should have called the parents into the staffroom to tell them about their children's problem…maybe some of us make the same mistake.

To this comment by Mr Owino, Mr Ndegwa perceptively replied, 'It happens!' This video and Mr Ndegwa's 'it happens' comment, verified pupils' claims that some teachers seldom maintained confidentiality, and frequently breached trust. Others, like Mr Owino, felt that the pupils in their acting had not portrayed teachers as 'serious enough' and thus made the learning process look frivolous, as presented in the conversation below:

Mr Owino:	Look, some pupils are not attentive and when the teacher is asking questions and points at them, they do not answer at all.
Interviewer:	Is that normal? Because they were supposed to show what happens in the class?
Mr Owino:	It happens, but they are supposed to raise up their hands and answer the questions! But in the video I see the pupils did not answer even one question!
Interviewer:	But is that normal in your classroom?
Mr Owino:	It is normal, it happens.

Mr Oile also complained about the teacher's behaviour in the same video, where the teacher was extremely friendly with the parents, greeting them with a local informal handshake: 'I would like to add an observation…especially the mode of greeting by the teacher to the parents…that one was not pleasing at all!' (The handshake involves slapping of the hands, a swaying of the body, and pressing each other's thumbs twice.)

The American scholar Charles Cooley would describe these teachers as peering through a 'looking glass self', a consequence of which led to some defensiveness. Cooley (1967) believed that the sense of self was not only formed by one's actual experiences, but also by imagining others' ideas of oneself. He explained that the self has three principal elements. The first step is that we imagine how we (and our actions) appear to other people. This is like getting a glimpse of ourselves as we would in a mirror. For example, going by the teachers' disappointments, it is likely that they thought of themselves as organised, authoritative and confidential. In the second step, we imagine how others judge us. For example, through the videos, it dawned on the teachers that the pupils had seen flaws in the teachers, something they were not pleased about. Cooley thus deduces that a person's self-concept is developed through the judgements of others – we come to see ourselves as we are influenced by what others say or think about us, and how we imagine others think of us. In this case, teachers put themselves through the looking glass and what emerges seems to bring some resolution.

Cognitive dissonance theory (Festinger 1957), which will be discussed later in this chapter, can also be used to understand teachers' reactions to sex education. In some cases, it is clear that what they thought of themselves, what parents and stakeholders thought of their teaching, and what their pupils thought of them caused conflict rather than resolution.

Teachers' challenges with the social spaces of HIV/AIDS education

The teacher-pupil and teacher-parent challenges raised during discussions about the video documentaries paved the way for further reflection on the challenges that our teachers faced when it came to HIV/AIDS and sex education in their schools. These challenges were similar in the three countries and are well documented among sub-Saharan scholars (see Altinyelken 2010; Kiragu 2007 and Njue et al. 2009). Some of these challenges have also been noted in the UK (see, for example, Blake 2002; Burbules & Hansen 1997 and Thomson & Scott 1992). These challenges include busyness, problems of language, a lack of guidelines, training and support from stakeholders, and the burden of being forced to act as a parent in the absence of parental interest. Each will be considered in turn.

Too much to do, too little time

Teachers reported that the mainstream curriculum was very demanding and required much more time than they had available in order to adequately prepare and deliver it. Many spoke of having to work 'overtime'. Core subjects like maths, science and English were given priority because they were known to be the most difficult for students. Consequently, HIV/AIDS education was relegated, especially since it was not examinable or enjoyable. Teachers frequently reported their unease with teaching on these culturally and religiously sensitive topics. They displayed their lack of confidence in talking to adolescents about HIV and sex, and described it as 'not an easy task' (Mr Ndegwa, School A, Kenya) and 'difficult and frightening' (Mr Ojwang, School B, Kenya). Teachers in Kenya and South Africa said they sometimes used role plays, poems and music to diffuse the awkwardness and embarrassment, yet still remained not completely at ease.

Lack of clear guidelines

Because there was no demarcated timetable slot or HIV/AIDS syllabus in most schools, it was not clear to teachers about when, how and what to teach on this topic. They also expressed anxiety about establishing the right level at which to pitch the subject in order to ensure it was both age- and gender-appropriate. Many spoke of how HIV and sex education was taught on an ad hoc basis. Ms Nafula (School A, Kenya) talked about having a problem in knowing what and how to teach the children in lower primary, and felt it was easier to talk to older pupils. South Africa has a dedicated learning area within which HIV/AIDS and sex education is to be taught (i.e. life orientation), but teachers in Kenya and Tanzania had to infuse or integrate HIV/AIDS education into their existing core subjects and other co-curricular activities. Examples of how they did this were presented in Chapter 4, and this included solving mathematical problems that included HIV statistics, reading and writing stories with an HIV theme in English and Swahili, and writing and performing songs and poems with an HIV focus in English and Swahili. In Tanzania, science was the primary 'carrier subject'. Consequently, because HIV/AIDS is taught from a biological perspective in science, the teacher is apt to teach facts on transmission rather than the emotional, social and relational dynamics of the pandemic.

In two schools in Kenya, although there were special education units that were meant to equip teachers for teaching HIV/AIDS education, many complained that their requests for help with dilemmas and issues, as described above, were ignored. All three methods of teaching HIV and sex education seemed to be flawed in each of the three countries. Infusing the subject meant it omitted central approaches to it. Having a special education unit meant to train teachers has failed in terms of reach. Having it as a stand-alone subject does not guarantee that it will be taught. Even in the presence of clear guidelines, some, such as Boler and Aggleton (2004), draw attention to the difficulty teachers face when they are expected to incorporate a different educational approach (in this case, one that is more participatory) into their pre-existing system (frequently teacher-driven and non-participatory).

Lack of training

Overall, teachers did not feel that they were adequately trained. For most, HIV/AIDS was an emerging phenomenon when they were in college and consequently it was not part of the training curriculum for them. When it was added, it was not taught in an in-depth manner owing to teacher trainers' lack of knowledge along with the widespread embarrassment and stigma that accompanied the disease at the time. Teachers talked of being trained for a single session ('one afternoon'), for several sessions as part of annual monitoring visits, or through short courses on integrating HIV/AIDS into the curriculum conducted by education ministries, departments or non-governmental organisations (NGOs). Ms Nyakio from School B in Kenya was among only a few teachers that spoke of the difference that this sort of training made. She had gone through several training workshops with local NGOs and said she felt 'more confident' in teaching HIV/AIDS education. She now served as the school's HIV/AIDS coordinator, leading the HIV club in the school and the in-service training for fellow teachers in the field. In contrast to Ms Nyakio's experience, Boler and Aggleton (2004) caution that in-service training is frequently ineffective because it is predominantly delivered through a 'cascade' approach. Such an approach is too superficial to allow meaningful learning to occur. Additionally, it is unrealistic to expect teachers to adapt to a different type of teaching while they remain within the confines of the same classroom, pressures and society. Instead, training must address each of these areas and be more comprehensive and in-depth than the usual 'cascade' approaches allow.

Owing to their lack of training, teachers faced dilemmas in the classroom when there was a pupil who was either infected or affected in the class. Their problem was how they could teach without hurting the feelings of such pupils, as described by Ms Makena, School C, Kenya:

> If you know the child's background…you should be careful when giving examples in class because the child may think you're personalising the issue and then he/she may not want to come to school when there's an HIV lesson…If you have an orphan you should not choose him as an example.

Language and the problem of sexual terminology

The language and discourse used in HIV/AIDS education was another challenge (Altinyelken 2010). Teachers reported their embarrassment and loss of dignity in not only having to use words like 'penis', 'vagina' and 'sex', but also talking about them in front of children. Ms Van Zyl from School B in South Africa spoke of her discomfort: 'The pupils challenge you. They want to hear those words come out of you, but unfortunately they then turn it around in their own little stories.' Ms Yeki from School A, South Africa, said that she used euphemisms, such as 'bhuti' (brother) for a penis, and 'sisi' (sister) for a vagina. Ms Dube, also from School A in South Africa, said that the problem lay with the teacher because most pupils she had taught 'do not have a problem [using the words]'. The giggles that ensued from the class when they did made it more difficult for them. However, Ms Tremain from School B in South Africa seemed to handle it well:

> Sometimes the minute you start talking about sex, the children start to laugh…They cut you off… sexual organs become a laughing matter…They want to paint a dirty picture to it. At this point you as a teacher feel that you don't want to talk about it. But on the other hand I explain that, 'You know that's what you have, that's what I have, and there is nothing funny about it. Why do you laugh when you say the word 'penis'? Why do you laugh when you say the word 'vagina'?' I try to stress that I have it, your mother has it, your father has it, and your grandfather has it, so we all have it. So please don't laugh…let's get on with the lesson!

The difficulty of being open and using sexual terms appropriately was heightened by the fact that some teachers had children, nephews, nieces or children of family friends in their classrooms, as observed by Mr Owino (School A, Kenya):

> You know some pupils are related to some teachers and some teachers feel that it is very hard to teach such a topic to the pupils. So culture is a factor preventing HIV/AIDS education to be taught the way it is supposed to be taught.

Helleve et al. (2009b) reported that teachers have contrasting views on teaching about sex and AIDS. Some of these concern cultural issues, but others see teaching these topics as a response to 'moral decline' among youth or 'teaching issues that parents failed to address'. Frequently, 'teachers were more concerned about young people's sexual behaviour than about preventing HIV/AIDS. They perceived that cultural contradictions between what was taught and local cultural values were an issue to which they needed to respond…Some took an adaptive approach to try to avoid conflicts, while others claimed the moral neutrality of their teaching.' (Helleve et al. 2009b: 189)

Dembélé and Lefoka (2007: 534) write about teachers having 'filters'. These are skills, beliefs, values and experiences that the teacher brings into the classroom, and which they had before becoming teachers. These filters determine their teaching practices and response to new ideas. As seen so far, one of these filters is silence on sexual issues and a belief that speaking about sex would lead children to early experimentation.

Lack of support from parents, the community and culture

A further challenge expressed by teachers involved negative reactions from parents, clergy and the local community. They feared that they would be accused of talking to children about sex and thus encouraging sexual activity. They also feared the stigma surrounding HIV and AIDS in their countries and understood that local communities chose silence as their preferred method to deal with it. Ms Yeki (School A, South Africa) summarised these fears:

> Because of this fear, I feel I am not teaching it in the way I would have liked. I can't go deep because if the learners talk about these things, parents are going to ask, 'Oh you have been taught that at school?' So it will sound like we are teaching children *amanyala* [taboo issues].

This further illustrates what has been discussed above regarding silence around sex as a filter teachers bring with them into the classroom. In addition, Ms Tremain (School B, South Africa) recalled how she had once taught in a rural school 'where it was totally taboo to talk about sex to children'. She added that although no one ever told her not to talk about sex, it was 'a silent unwritten contract' in the community not to do so.

Ms Papier (School B, South Africa) also said that her problem had been when she taught her pupils 'one thing in school and they get something else at home'. This created dissonance in the child. Ms Papier continued to describe her frustration at the current state of affairs: 'Sometimes you feel like you are hitting your head against the wall because you don't get support from home or parents.' She related an example in which a parent, described as a devoted Christian and who, because her Christian beliefs, would not allow her daughter to wear trousers, came to the school to challenge the teacher over her teaching of sex education:

> This mother came to the school and said she did not like what she heard from her child. I told her this is the way our children live these days. We must not avoid these things [sex]…or the child will hear from their peers while you as a teacher will be careful when saying those things.

Mr Oile, School A, Kenya, concurred: 'There is silence in the home and that is where this thing [sex] takes place…We are trying but we are failed by the parents.' Kiragu (2009) describes Mr Oile and Ms Papier's dilemmas as having a 'heavy tongue'. In both cases, these teachers are aware of the dilemma, but feel compelled (through fear of parental censure) not to even use the word sex, replacing it instead with 'things' or 'thing'. Though they teach in different countries, these teachers face similar challenges. In Tanzania, Mr Jecha, School C, talked of how one parent had stormed into school with a science textbook, claiming that children were too young to be taught about HIV/AIDS issues in class three (nine years old). He described the parent as being 'furious and claimed that we had been teaching the children immoral things'. Female teachers were also concerned about their reputation, as seeming to know about sex was regarded as an unfeminine quality, a view supported by Campbell (2003), and described by Ms Kwamboka, School C, Kenya:

> Mostly Africans say that if a woman usually talks about sex education they think you are street woman…In some communities if a teacher likes to teach about sex education they will say you are a manner-less teacher.

In contrast to this fear of parents and the antagonism shown by parents, a few teachers described parents who were grateful that the teacher talked to their child because they (parents) were too shy to do it. Ms Kerubo, a head teacher from School C in Kenya, recollected how one parent had thanked her for telling her child 'everything'. However, for this head teacher, 'everything' did not include information about same-sex relationships. Ms Nyawira, also from School C, Kenya, talked about gay relationships. Both teachers labelled it as 'sodomy':

> I chased two boys from the school because if the teacher starts the lesson they will go to the toilet and do nasty things and I could not allow such a thing and even the education officer came to follow up and I asked her, 'Can you allow your child to be sodomised?' I suggested to her that the boys should not stay together but for her to recommend they go to different schools and she wrote the letter. (Ms Kerubo, School C, Kenya)

> There is this boy I used to teach in another school who used to teach other boys about sodomy. He was eight years old and I sent him to call his mother. The following day his mother did not come so I sent his older sister to call her and when she came back she told me that her mother said it is normal. Later I came to realise that his Madrasa [religious school] teacher used to molest him. To them it was just normal. If that teacher is HIV-positive he will be spreading it to the children. (Ms Nyawira, School C, Kenya)

The cases above exemplify Kehily's (2002: 53) argument of a normative heterosexuality in the schools' discourse. She says that 'the processes of dominant practice, school routines and procedures situated within the curriculum and pedagogic practice…serve to shape and consolidate heterosexual relations. If sex is discussed at all in schools, it is assumed to be normatively heterosexual.' In Kenya, as in a number of other African countries, same-sex relationships remain criminalised. This complicates the sexual discourse in schools, which while aiming at a human rights discourse must contend both with the existing legal framework and the religious and cultural taboos opposing same-sex relationships.

The *in loco parentis* role

To deal with some of the challenges that HIV/AIDS had presented to their pupils and families, teachers literally took up an *in loco parentis* role (Latin for 'in the place of a parent'). They spoke about how the burden of HIV/AIDS and sex education fell on them. Many of their pupils were orphaned and vulnerable, having lost one or both parents to HIV/AIDS. Some were now carers to their sibling and/or a sick relative.

Ms Kerubo, the head teacher of School C, Kenya, talked about how a member of the school committee, a widower, had 10 children to look after, after losing three of his brothers to AIDS. At times the other committee members contributed money to help him shoulder the burden, but it was never enough. In the same school, some children attended school for a half day and spent the other half in town selling groundnuts or boiled maize to survive. Hunt (2009) talks about how child labour is either enabling for education if the money earned is used for schooling, or is disenabling if the money is not invested in the child's schooling. In our study both nutrition and school attendance suffered because the money earned by these children hardly met their daily needs.

Ms Kerubo also told researchers how they had lost 'a bright girl' this way. Her family circumstances forced her to drop out of school and enter a life of commercial sex work in order to survive. AIDS has led to poor school attendance and retention. Teachers are in the position of having to deal with these children in the absence of parents, or in cases where the parents are debilitated. Teachers were also emotionally affected when some of their learners died of HIV/AIDS or drug-related circumstances, as reported in Kenya and South Africa. Ms Carpenter from South Africa said, 'One of my former students had stopped taking drugs a few months ago, but it was too late. He died on Friday. I could not believe it because he was young…I mean…it so sad.' Teachers frequently saw their role in providing sex and HIV/AIDS education as a parental duty in order to prevent children from having to experience some of the dire consequences of the condition. They do this despite opposition from parents.

Separation of sexual knowledges acquired in and out of school

Another challenge flagged by teachers was the quite considerable insulation and contradictions between what the teachers taught in HIV/AIDS education and the children's lives outside of school. Ms Papier (School B, South Africa) was disturbed that she taught about abstinence and fidelity, and yet some of her pupils 'have got different fathers…he has a child in each avenue…the mothers have got different partners, and they are all one big family'. Teachers reported that many children got to know about their step-siblings at school through rumours and gossip. Ms Scott from School B, South Africa, also described how her pupils 'see and hear sex every day in their homes, as families have limited living space and therefore no privacy'. She said that as a consequence, it was not uncommon for some pupils who were brothers and sisters to start having sex with each other at puberty. This reflects the acts of incest that Trevor, a pupil from South Africa, spoke about in Chapter 5. Ms Scott felt that children were having problems knowing what was right because what happened at home was the opposite of what was taught in school. Even advising children to avoid teenage pregnancy was a problem because numerous children had teenage mothers, as she describes:

> The other day I was shocked when one of my pupils invited me to her mother's 21st birthday, and I said, 'No, your mother can never be 21 and you are six years!' The next Tuesday was a parents' day and her mommy came and I told her her child [had] invited me to her birthday. And she confirmed that she was turning 21…So you can imagine…that means her mother got pregnant at age 15. (Ms Scott, School B, South Africa)

Mr Manage from School C, Tanzania, and Ms Kerubo from School C, Kenya, also gave examples of how factors from outside the school contradicted what they taught in HIV/AIDS education in school, especially with regard to topics such as pornography, prostitution/gift sex and religion. She described another example – kesha has already been mentioned – about religious practice paradoxically facilitating sexual activity:

> I think Islam encourages premarital sex because there is a certain time girls are taken to an old lady who teaches them how to handle their man, how to play the game [have sex]…There was a time a number of Muslim girls did not turn up [to school] for a week and when they came back I asked one

of them where they had been and she told me they had gone…to an old lady…who taught them how to please their husbands. Once they are taught, they will want to practise and they are only 11 to 12 years. (Ms Kerubo, School C, Kenya)

Several scholars would dispute Ms Kerubo's thoughts and argue that such sex education is deeply rooted in pre-colonial traditions and provides a safe space where girls learn about sexuality and pleasure from an older, experienced and trusted community member (see Bryk 1933; Jeater 1993 and Kenyatta 1938 for examples from Uganda, Zimbabwe and Kenya, respectively). Even with such explicit teachings, teenage sex and pregnancy were not common in pre-colonial times. These teachings also contrast with the current resistance to any consideration of sexual pleasure in school-based HIV/AIDS education. However, it is worth noting that Ms Kerubo's example is limited to girls learning how to please men; it is perhaps rarely ever the other way round. This is an example of 'the missing discourse of female desire' described by Fine (1988: 35). Fine observes that a discourse of female desire, pleasure or sexual entitlement is missing and that as a result women struggle to untangle issues of gender, power and the constrictions of a male-defined sexuality. Tepper (2000: 288) affirms that 'sexuality as a source of pleasure and as an expression of love is not readily recognised [and is under-represented in literature] for populations that have been traditionally marginalised in society such as women…and children'. This clash between teaching an empowering sexuality, especially for young women, and teaching no sex at all in school is an enormous and ongoing problem in the school context.

In addressing the general gap between pupils' knowledge from in and out of school, Mr Matu from School C, Kenya, described in detail how he attempts to bridge this gap and understand pupils' experiences and problems:

Last year when I was a class teacher of class 8, there was a boy and a girl who would dash home every lunchtime. In the afternoon they would be sleepy in class and at times they would not come back. When I sat and talked to some of their classmates they told me, 'Teacher they always go home to have sex over lunchtime and then come back in the afternoon.'…I realised that in this school, children are very exposed. I now make an effort to talk to pupils. At times I take a walk to the bus stop with them after class…we just walk and have an open discussion and they will tell me, 'Teacher so and so is pregnant, so and so's mother has HIV.'…So I come to learn more about them. I now talk to them at least on a weekly basis or daily if it is possible…When I am teaching I will go and sit in the seat next to the child…I lower myself to their level. I do not want them to look at me as a teacher who is at a distance. Let them look at me as a parent, a brother…that is the way I can get information from them. I know I will be able to save a few before they get to the point of no return.

Pierre Bourdieu (1989: 16) in describing the elements of social space and its structures writes:

People who are very distant from each other in social space can encounter one another and interact, if only briefly and intermittently, in physical space. Interactions…mask the structures that are realized in them. This is one of those cases where the visible, that which is immediately given, hides the invisible which determines it. One thus forgets that the truth of any interaction is never entirely to be found within the interaction as it avails itself for observation.

Bourdieu would describe Mr Matu as a teacher trying to unmask prevalent structures, 'where the visible, that which is immediately given' – for example the pupils' truancy – 'hides the invisible which determines it' (i.e. that they were having sex). His caution is that we should not forget that 'the truth of any interaction is never entirely to be found within the interaction as it avails itself for observation'. Most importantly, Bourdieu theorises regarding Mr Matu removing social space between children and teachers – a theme to which we will later return.

Summarising teachers' consultations: Looking-glass experience

In our study, we found that teachers were aware and critical of their own practice. Though some were more open than others in terms of talking about sex, most found themselves using a protective discourse when it came to teaching HIV/AIDS education. They felt embarrassed and incapable of being open about sexual matters, with many using euphemisms for sexual terms. This was despite being aware of their pupils' sexualised out-of-school world. It points to the power of sociocultural aspects of silence, taboo and stigma where sexual issues are concerned. Teachers further spoke about their challenges in teaching about HIV/AIDS, some which were technical in nature, such as lack of training, struggles to implement syllabus guidelines, and manage resources and time, while others were sociocultural (or socio-historical), such as fearing parents and the gap between what they taught and what they knew was happening in homes. Tabulawa (1997: 192) writes that approaching teachers' problems as only technical in nature – and hence attempting to solve them through interventions such as teacher in-service programmes, workshops and seminars, all aimed at changing the teacher's classroom behaviour – has had little impact in the classroom, as evidenced in our study. Consequently, the teacher is blamed directly for any failures. But there are other wider social contexts that act as filters and influence the locus of pedagogical change because pedagogical views are socially and historically grounded (Tabulawa 1997). For example, most countries in Africa still operate within the bureaucratic and authoritative climate inherited from the missionary/colonial era, and are also influenced by African traditional culture where the adult is seen as having more wisdom than the child. Sex, a taboo topic in many cultures, also limits teachers' freedom to teach sex education and influences their way of teaching it. Understanding these sociocultural determinants to pedagogy may help shift blame from teachers, and concentrate on giving them support as well as addressing these complexities. Teachers' recognition of these challenges and shortcomings, however, is good news for change.

Community stakeholders' perceptions of HIV/AIDS education

Having discussed both learners' and teachers' perceptions about the HIV/AIDS education received and offered in the school, we now present community stakeholders' views. These are based on interviews conducted with approximately six stakeholders identified per school.

Studies conducted in developed countries indicate a strong positive correlation between parental involvement in sexuality education and the sexual health and awareness of adolescents (Aved & Zones 1985; Campbell & MacPhail 2002). Parents who communicate freely about sex and contraception have been found, for example, to have a significant influence on their children's decisions to use condoms (Aggleton & Campbell 2000). The degree to which young people feel their parents are concerned about their welfare is another factor that has been linked to them practising safe sex (Aggleton & Campbell 2000). However, previous research in South Africa (Campbell & MacPhail 2002; Francis 2010; Zisser & Francis 2006), in Kenya (Njue et al. 2009) and in Tanzania (Mkumbo & Ingham 2010) has emphasised adolescents' uneasiness about communicating with their parents about sex. In Campbell and MacPhail's (2000) study in a community near Johannesburg, youth interviewees stated that parents simply did not broach the subject; for these young people initiating such a discussion, on the other hand, would signify 'lack of respect' (Campbell & MacPhail 2002: 21). Prazak (2000: 83) also notes how 'relationships of respect' hinder communication on sexuality in Kuria District, Kenya.

The data collected from interviews conducted in Kenyan, South African and Tanzanian communities presents the range of attitudes towards sex education for youth, from dismay at its perceived negative effects to confidence in its ability to curtail HIV/AIDS infections. The observations made in the literature regarding the lack of parental involvement nevertheless reflect strongly most parents' and community members' responses to questions posed to them in this study. The evidence also points to something more than just a disconnect between young people and sceptical parents and grandparents in the three countries. Notably, several participants registered a distinct sense of internal conflict – they acknowledged the benefits of HIV/AIDS education in schools and admitted knowing that they should communicate more openly with their children, but simultaneously gave a reason for why they were not able to do so. Griffiths et al. (2008: 719) refer to individuals experiencing this personal struggle as being in a state of 'emotional and informational conflict'. Cognitive dissonance theory provides a useful tool by which to engage analytically with this sense of internal tension, and will be discussed shortly.

Does sex education encourage sex?

The second major theme to emerge in parents' and community members' attitudes towards HIV/AIDS education was the concern that young people would interpret advice on condom use as encouraging them to have sex. As Campbell and MacPhail (2002: 21) note of the South African context, '[s]tudies…have reported that apart from feeling embarrassed to discuss sex with their children, parents often believe that discussion of contraception will encourage their children to become sexually active'. Similar reports have emerged from Kenya (Njue et al. 2009) and Tanzania (Mkumbo & Ingham 2010). This apprehension that HIV/AIDS education hastens sexual debut or increases sexual behaviour is a common perception of HIV/AIDS-education programmes worldwide (Aggleton & Crewe 2005; Ryan 1989). The conclusion of Kirby et al. (2006) in their analysis of 83 assessments of sex- and HIV-education programmes targeted at youth is particularly striking, therefore, for its unequivocal stance that the programmes did not increase or initiate sexual activity. In contrast, they found that many of the initiatives, including some based in Kenya, South Africa and Tanzania, had the opposite effect and in fact 'delayed or reduced sexual activity either among the entire sample or important sub-groups within the sample' (Kirby et al. 2006: 45). To be sure, a number of community-stakeholder respondents in each country, several of whom were directly involved in school structures, were unequivocally supportive of school-based HIV/AIDS education. However, the comprehensive review of Kirby et al. (2006) prompts the question, why did many parents and community members interviewed in this study express such vehement and negative views on HIV/AIDS education, which promotes condom use as best sexual practice? Respondents' perceptions were couched variously in religious and cultural modes, but almost always in moral imperatives that suggested a generational disconnect, as if something in society had 'broken' so that discipline among young people was a thing of the past.

Why do parents and other adults feel uncomfortable about HIV/AIDS education?

We will now turn to the apparent discomfort with which certain individuals perceived and explained their role in educating young people about sex and HIV/AIDS. It is useful to consider what alternative cognitions or 'traits a person knows about himself, and about his surroundings' (Mwale 2009: 461) in order to understand the strategies respondents employed in order to offset the dissonance of harbouring conflicting ideas of HIV/AIDS education. The two overarching ideas that seemed to strike the greatest discord among interviewees, especially in South Africa, were, firstly, the need to raise awareness among young people about HIV/AIDS and safe sex through school-based education and parent-child communication, and, secondly, the notion that a person's culture either implicitly or explicitly constrains one from talking about sexuality.

Cognitive dissonance and culture

According to cognitive dissonance theory, '[d]issonance is a negative drive or state of "psychological discomfort or tension", which motivates people to reduce it by achieving consonance' (Mwale 2009: 461). In this sense, several South African parents' continual reference to their culture appears as an alternative cognition in itself, one which frees them of the responsibility to communicate with their children. Therefore, a South African nurse (identified from School A) states, 'Like the way we black people have been brought up, it is difficult to be exposed to sexual orientation.' She continues, 'Our mindset is still in the old order, the way our parents brought us up, we are also doing the same thing with our children; people of my generation are still not free to talk with our children.'

Another illustrative example of the way in which interviewees' sense of culture was expressed as a constraint from participating in any aspect of HIV/AIDS education is seen in a statement by a South African grandparent (School A) that she does not discourage her granddaughter's attendance at loveLife programmes (a major South African youth sex-education programme) because 'she needs to know [about sexuality] and we older people are still embarrassed to talk about it, although we are encouraged to talk about it'. Although her upbringing made her 'scared to talk about sex', the grandparent acknowledged that 'AIDS affects old people irrespective of their culture'. By shifting the responsibility of sex education onto loveLife, she is able to avoid the taboo topic of sex without discarding her view that 'it is not wise for people not to talk openly about this thing because it destroys everybody, even a parent because when a child is sick it affects the parents as well'.

The above example provides an instance of an individual attempting to disentangle herself from her own 'emotional and informational conflict' by entrusting an external role player with the job of teaching young people, and so ties in with the way the school emerged in many interviews as the primary forum for HIV/AIDS education. For example, a South African parent stated, 'You see, it is better now with the school, because a child hears about something at school and they will say it bluntly to a parent. You cannot say, "No, where did you hear about that?" You have to give them answers. So the teachers are helping us since we are not open about these things.'

Moral and generational concerns

Although perceptions of culture informed a number of interviewees' responses to HIV/AIDS and sex education, in some instances, the discourse on culture as an obstacle to communication was extended so that it reflected moral and generational concerns that were very often intertwined. For example, a South African traditional healer (School A) claimed black people have undermined their culture to the extent that they now 'follow the culture of the whites'. He continued, 'We have nothing of our own we can be proud of as we were in the old days. We are just like people who adopt a culture that is not ours.' At the heart of this traditional healer's grievances is his view that in following 'white culture', levels of discipline among young people have dropped. He states, 'I don't consider AIDS as an aspect of our culture, I consider it as something that came up since we abandoned our customs.' In a similar vein, a Kenyan male elder bluntly asserted, 'The environment has no discipline.'

This view of pervasive moral degradation permeates the interviews, and there is a strong sense that parents, grandparents and religious leaders perceive a world in which they are losing their grip on authority and social stability: things are not what they ought to be. Thus one finds a South African nurse asserting that 'these days the youth have changed their behaviour, I can say they are crazy about sex'. Similarly, two mothers interviewed together in Kenya recounted a 15-year-old's descent into drugs and prostitution as an example of the way in which the youth no longer pay heed to adults. Included in their allegations was the statement that young people 'talk very bad…[and] even attack you' if confronted by an elder. While elements of their assertions are undoubtedly true, from this blanket perspective 'precocious sexual activity' (Aggleton & Crewe 2005: 303) among youth is to be both expected and deplored as a generational flaw. Finally, a school committee member from School B, Tanzania, described a situation in an area in Dar es Salaam in which 'most of the parents are not stable [attentive] with their children'. The respondent explained what was meant by stability:

> That causes for the bad behaviours learned by children, we can say a child is behaving like a domestic fowl, that is when leaving home in the morning, no one cares whether the child has returned home or not. And when the child does not want to go to school, the parent is not asking for reasons and therefore in the end a child maybe picking up scrap metals for sale.

In contrast to the previous accusations made against youth immorality, here the blame for societal degradation sits with parents. The speaker nonetheless indicates that young people's behaviour is abnormal and casts youth as being outside of bounded norms. The implicit message is that young people's actions cannot be monitored and an inevitable process begins:

> You will find that teenage students in the neighbourhood tend to attend those parties which are meaningless. By doing so that child will be affected by all evil happening in that party. In the end you will be having a school-absconding child or maybe a prostitute before maturity due to peer pressure. Hence then, you can be having HIV/AIDS education but still be ineffective due to those environmental factors. (School C committee member, Tanzania)

As salient as culture and morality proved to be in determining interviewees' attitudes towards HIV/AIDS education, especially in the South African context, the Tanzanian example was distinctive in that respondents frequently went beyond identifying cultural practices as a challenge to communicating about sex. Several individuals singled out female genital mutilation as antithetical to attempts to reduce instances of HIV/AIDS infection.

Mkumbo and Ingham (2010), in their study of 287 Tanzanian parents' views on sex education, conclude that 75 per cent of respondents supported school-based instruction. One might tentatively draw parallels between their study and the striking difference between responses provided by Tanzanians in the present study. A statement by a Kenyan female elder further revealed the way in which perceptions of culture can vary vastly between people and across borders:

> You know, [in the] old times our parents used to educate us, but nowadays parents don't have time. They say they will learn from school, they will see on TV. They leave to others to do it. You, the parents, should teach your children, as we used to be told.

Her statement evokes a better tradition of education that has since been forgotten. Its place has been filled instead by a modern and, she suggests, inadequate syllabus.

Religious obstacles

In some instances respondents' religious beliefs also surfaced as a challenge to the orthodox call for sexuality education. To quote a Tanzanian male parent, 'Truly, the way I see it…the teachings of the HIV/AIDS education in schools is good but it is going against the religious morals/ethics.' His words express a personal dilemma, but they also exemplify in stark terms a central question in HIV/AIDS education: how should one reconcile individuals' religious beliefs with the tenets of mainstream HIV/AIDS education? Is it at all possible to do so?

The disjuncture between religion and orthodox education was most apparent in discussions on safe sex. Conservative Muslims and Christians frequently maintained that advocating condom use encouraged sex among the youth. Abstinence, they insisted, is both safer and morally correct. According to a Christian-religion teacher (Mr John, School A, Tanzania), 'a student should not use a condom because…first of all the condom makes him/her fail to control themselves…his/her temptations'. An Islamic male elder (School C, Kenya) had similar views and used bread and butter as metaphors for sex and condoms, as seen in the following conversation:

Islamic elder: Talking depends on how you approach it. Like you tell them this action [sex] you are not allowed to do. Don't tell them to use a condom. When you tell somebody don't take the bread without butter they will try to take bread alone, thus it leads to same thing. Why tell somebody, do this with this [have sex with a condom], rather than don't do it?

Interviewer:	You don't see that telling the person to take bread and butter as saving a life?
Islamic elder:	No, if the bread is bad, say the bread is finished!
Interviewer:	You know how some children are? When you tell them not to eat bread that is when they eat it all the more. Maybe that bread and butter saves lives?
Islamic elder:	I don't see it like that! Sometimes you have to use force to push. If you want a child to listen you have to push…you punish them not to hurt them but discipline them. We need to teach them not to do this [have sex] and I tell them not to use these things [condoms]. Only adults should know about condoms.

An Islamic religion teacher from Kenya summed up the dilemma, referring to differing sources of authority, and argued, 'Everyone has a book which is guidance…We Muslims have a book and our colleagues have their book which is their guidance. So that which is in their books is what they should follow.' He might just as easily have been referring to school authorities and their textbooks, as opposed to the texts of other religions.

A theoretical analysis and practical solution

The responses of these religious teachers and elders evoke a pedagogy of the past, which Bernstein (1996: 66) terms a 'retrospective pedagogic identity', in which grand narratives of the past 'are appropriately recontextualised to stabilise that past in the future'. As one manifestation of this retrospective identity, Bernstein (1996: 75) suggests a 'fundamentalist' mode, which 'provides for an unambiguous, stable, intellectually impervious, collective identity'. In the context of perceived immorality and changes in the hierarchies of religious and cultural authority, it is not difficult to see how such a pedagogical identity might be invoked by those in a position to do so. In that the knowledge and criteria for belonging to a retrospective identity are based on a core narrative, it opposes any extraneous information as illegitimate and delivers a centralised, top-down message to its audience. From the standpoint of sex education, the pitfalls of such an approach become immediately evident. As Allen (2007: 221) notes of New Zealand schools, the official discourses contained in sexuality education 'work to simultaneously acknowledge student sexuality and position young people as "childlike"'. She contends that young people are disenfranchised to the point that 'schools can be seen to undermine the kind of sexual agency that young people might access to support their sexual well-being' (Allen 2007: 221). Similarly, Francis (2010: 315) advocates recognising young people as 'knowers', a stance which, she argues, 'challenges the idea that sexuality is something that can be handed to youth in appropriate doses'.

When a community decries a school's attempts to educate children on condom use as encouraging sexual behaviour, as one Kenyan school chairperson described, it not only stakes its confidence in abstinence alone, but also reveals its reluctance to attribute children with the ability to make informed decisions. Francis's notion of young people as 'knowers' challenges such an attitude entirely. When children's parents are unwilling to talk about sexuality, especially considering they almost certainly did not receive formalised sex education themselves, the task of changing this attitude is arguably a difficult one. Indeed, the undertaking would be made even more challenging if a religious or cultural fundamentalist attitude prevails. To turn the situation on its head, however, parents' unwillingness to communicate, either because of fear or discomfort, might perhaps be exactly the point at which educators could broach the impasse. The notion of a decentralised classroom, which would espouse the opposite principles to a retrospective pedagogical approach – one that longs for the past – would arguably satisfy Allen's call to empower youth. Instead of withholding or discounting unauthorised experiences, such an approach would encourage learning outside of official spaces.

Two studies seeking to test precisely the sort of egalitarian mode discussed above are useful to consider. The first, a 1996 pilot scheme designed by Oliver, Leeming and Dwyer (1998), provides an example of what an integrated, decentralised sexuality-education programme might look like. The study involved grade 5–8 students in Tennessee and sought to expand the ambit of school-based sex education so that, through joint homework tasks, parents would actively participate in their child's learning process. The clear benefit of such an approach is that it addresses the generational gap between parent and child. If the chronic lack of communication on sexuality is, as we suggest, due to a disconnect between young people and adults, then mutual learning must be the first step towards a common understanding. The second study is Orner's (1996) investigation into what she terms 'situated pedagogy'. The author's central thesis is that intervention projects, which put young people in positions to address topics in their immediate environment, are able to 'intervene in culture through education' and 'intervene in education through the production of culture' (Orner 1996: 73). In short, the projects challenge the top-down approach to education, which typically addresses students more as an audience than as individual actors embedded in 'myriad political, social, and cultural struggles' (Orner 1996: 72). In many ways, Orner's situated pedagogy is one that generates new knowledge as much as it is informed by any officially sanctioned syllabus. Throughout our study, by consulting pupils about HIV/AIDS education we have attempted to achieve a similar egalitarian mode. By including parents and other adult stakeholders, we attempt to take concerns about religion, culture and morality seriously without excluding the needs of children and the science that shows that HIV/AIDS education does not increase sexual experimentation.

All that is left to address, perhaps, is the question of how to resolve tensions between religion and mainstream sex-education approaches. Health communication scholars have questioned whether theories of communication for behaviour change that focus primarily on the individual are as widely applicable as has previously been assumed. Airhihenbuwa and Obregon (2000: 5) specifically argue that culture, often noted by researchers and practitioners for its muffling effects on communication, 'should be viewed for its strength and not always as a barrier'. This standpoint reflects calls made by interviewees, especially religious leaders, with strong religious beliefs for school-based sex education to be sensitive to religious beliefs. This view is encapsulated in a comment made by a Christian-religion teacher from Tanzania:

> I would ask that the seminars [held by the government] should bring us together. Because you find that only the teachers of the schools are called to seminars. But those children are taught by all of us and these religious teachers may then have challenges…they may see that in this thing we should do this…and in this we should do this. Finally when we come out we may resemble each other in certain aspect or we may differ in small area.

According to the integrative, decentralised model of consultative education proposed in this book, such appeals can and should be accommodated. To be sure, a holistic approach that recognises the nuances and sensitivities of different religions and cultures will inevitably provide more comprehensive information for young people to draw on and form an understanding of their own sexuality. And ultimately, once officially sanctioned information is taken down from its pedestal and hierarchies of knowledge are abolished, young people will then be properly empowered to make informed and cogent decisions. In offering the points of view they have in this chapter, they show themselves to be eminently capable of doing so.

Reflections on social space

This chapter has presented the voices of all our study participants, and the views of pupils, teachers and community stakeholders about the HIV/AIDS and sex education taught in the school. Through videos, pupils communicated that they currently received a teacher-driven, fact-based HIV/AIDS education, and yet what they wanted was one that was participatory, consultative, open and in-depth. Teachers affirmed what pupils said about current HIV/AIDS education – although there were a few who tried to be open about sexuality. Teachers articulated numerous challenges to their practice, and mostly identified technical and social issues that impeded their complete participation in HIV/AIDS-education delivery. Community stakeholders, though supportive of HIV/AIDS education in the school, felt that it should be taught within the confines of a protective discourse. Constant in all this is the teacher, who has to teach the curriculum.

Since HIV/AIDS education provides a 'social vaccine' effective in fighting HIV/AIDS, as discussed in Chapter 1, the role of the teacher is even more crucial. Teachers have an opportunity more than the other agents to bring about change because they are the ones who teach. Furthermore, they function as the glue that brings together pupils and stakeholders in this change process. But for them to bring about change, in this case change to their pedagogical approach, as pupils have requested, they too have to change. This is not easy, as they already have existing filters (Dembélé & Lefoka 2007) and are agents in a pre-established social space which has structural constraints that will influence the construction of their vision of the world. Bourdieu (1989) describes this as the 'habitus'. This social space is constructed in such a way that the closer the agents, groups or institutions are situated within a space, the more common properties they have – and vice versa. This theoretical construction is reflected in our data, where there was more homogeneity in the views of similar agents than in views from across the different participant groups. Nevertheless, even among similar agents, there can be different or antagonistic points of view. For example, in contrast to the majority, some teachers, like Ms Tremain from School B, South Africa, and some stakeholders, like the grandparent from South Africa who allowed her granddaughter to attend loveLife programmes, believed in being more open about sexuality, and even in talking about condoms or mentioning words like sex, vagina and penis.

As Bourdieu (1989: 19) describes it:

> [Habitus] is both a system of schemes of production of practices and a system of perception and appreciation of practices…And, in both of these dimensions, its operation expresses the social position in which it was elaborated. Consequently, habitus produces practices and representations which are available for classification, which are objectively differentiated; however, they are immediately perceived as such only by those agents who possess the code…to understand their social meaning. Habitus thus implies a 'sense of one's place' but also a 'sense of the place of others'.

Therefore, if teachers and stakeholders are to understand the children's world, they must strive to understand their pupils'/children's codes and habitus. This would involve a consultation of pupils, which is discussed in Chapter 7. However, it is a challenge for teachers to adopt a consultative approach because they have been used to following a didactic, non-participatory approach (Boler & Aggleton 2004). Using a language that pupils would understand is also imperative to improving teaching and learning. Dembélé and Lefoka (2007) suggest the implementation of bilingual education, whereby the home language – the language most familiar to the child – is used as an additional language, especially with small children. This is also true of sex and HIV/AIDS education – both figuratively and literally. These strategies of pedagogical and curricular renewal are expounded further in Chapters 7 and 8.

CHAPTER 7

Dialogues for change

In the previous chapters we have seen the complexity of educating children and young people about sexual matters clearly laid out. The cultural tensions are evident and the complex work of the teacher, who has to bridge the values and processes of the school community and the faster-moving world of young people, is manifest. We have also seen that young people are perceptive and notice almost all aspects of the sexual lives of the adults in their community; that they are keen to engage with adults in discussing and making sense of their experiences; and that they welcome active engagement in sex-education classes on HIV-related matters. We have seen the silence around sexuality and HIV/AIDS, and the ambiguity surrounding policy and practice. How then can one constructively engage with these dilemmas and tensions? Our hypothesis was that we might be able to achieve this through a dialogue between the actors: community members, teachers and pupils. In this chapter we explore the last phase of the research, which was a dialogue between the actors. The dialogues for change consisted of presenting the findings of the consultations with the children to all actors and discussing what the perceived implications were for action and transformation. The chapter first explores the idea of dialogue and its importance in education, before considering the various themes that emerged in these dialogues.

Dialogue – Its importance and process

The notion of dialogue as being central to education and knowledge creation is not a new one: Plato (Plato & Grube 2002) in his representation of Socrates in his writings argued that dialogue was the highest form of teaching and the path to knowledge. Plato argued that truth could be uncovered through a process of leading another through the steps and this was the role of the teacher. This view of dialogue as arriving at a fixed point is not the one being used here. The view we adopt is a more open-ended conception and more akin to that of Freire and Burbules. Freire (1970, 1985) made dialogue central to his discussion of the 'pedagogy of the oppressed'. In a later paper (Shor & Freire 1987: 14), he argued:

> Dialogue is the sealing together of the teacher and students in the joint act of knowing and re-knowing the object of study…instead of transferring the knowledge *statically*, as a *fixed possession of the teacher*, dialogue demands a dynamic approximation towards the object.

Freire's conception of dialogue is of a process that aims at the mutual development of understanding through a process of shared inquiry; it aims to empower the less powerful and it is seen as a process of enablement (Burbules 1993: 6). Whether this is a process of arriving at a preconceived point has been debated, but that was not our intention. The intended goal was to explore the possibility of arriving at a position of more mutual understanding. We have adopted the core aspects of Burbules's (1993) definition of dialogue. He argues that dialogue is *pedagogical* in that it is directed towards discovery and new understanding, which stands to improve the knowledge, insight or sensitivity of its participants (Burbules 1993: 8). Dialogue has a *moral* dimension (Bridges 1988), in that there is a value-based dimension to group discussion aiming at reaching a good and helpful outcome, and it is *constructivist*, in that it tries to build on what people already know. It is a *process of communication* that is linked to the 'values of involvement, respect and concern for one's partner' (Burbules 1993: 12) and, as such, is linked to democratic or egalitarian values. These particular and focused intentions make it different from a conversation or a group discussion.

In the course of our consultations with pupils, community members and teachers, we received theoretical knowledge from our participants. The consultations identified different and sometimes conflicting views on sex education, as well as on the position of adults in educating young people on sexual matters. The consultations revealed social tensions in teaching and learning about sex, and differing notions of the sexual knowledge young people had or should have, as well as how this should be regulated. There was not a fit in all cases between what the young people knew and wanted and what the adults wanted to give or thought appropriate. The idea of learning as scaffolding has been discussed, and this is, as Burbules (1993) points out, a fundamental notion related to how we change our minds or learn. It is based on the idea that we cannot change other people: they alone can change their minds or their decisions. We can engage in a dialogue, but not 'hand over' knowledge. Therefore, we believed that we could not merely instruct or tell adults to change their ways of working in matters of sexuality and HIV-related education – it would have little impact. However, the gap between the informal and formal knowledge that the children in our study displayed is a significant problem. So we wanted to explore what the reaction would be to engaging in a dialogue around the data. We were acting on the belief that this problem could not be resolved as an intellectual or research endeavour alone, but by working to establish more and better communication between the actors and addressing the serious institutional, generational and prejudicial barriers on both sides.

Impediments to dialogue

There were significant impediments to this dialogue. There were widely differing views on both sexuality education and the rights to knowledge of young people. The data had already shown that there was a desire for silence – there was silence from many adults around sexual matters for children – and yet the children wanted dialogue and active engagement with the issues. There was a pedagogy that, on the whole, was not constructivist, and the fundamental conceptions about learning, authority and the role of teachers and pupils were not widely shared. There were different languages used to speak about sexual matters and there was cultural diversity. There were also issues of power and voice. In both of these the role of gender was central.

There was not a long tradition of young people expressing their views on their learning; some of the teachers too were not necessarily used to speaking freely and openly about matters of teaching and learning. The conceptions of learning that we had seen, and particularly learning in the area of HIV/ AIDS, were that fear was a good teacher, as was information giving. Our data were challenging these ideas, as well as the fundamental idea of children as sexually innocent and in primary need of protection. Given these significant potential impediments and the scale and nature of the task we were keen to see how the dialogues would fare.

Dialogue of actors

As a starting point for the dialogues that were organised in each country (see Appendix 1 for the questions and process), we processed the data we have presented in the preceding chapters, and produced a sample of the photos that the young people had taken in the three countries. We analysed the interview data thematically so that we could present the main sources and content of young people's sexual knowledge and included this in our presentation. Finally, we showed edited versions of the video documentaries pupils had made to show the sort of sexuality- and HIV-related education that they would like. We invited four to six community members (including the ones that we had interviewed earlier in the process), four to six teachers from each school and four to six pupils who had participated in the research study from each school. In addition to the prime purpose of seeing what would happen when all participants engaged in the dialogue and understood each other's positions, we were aiming to find out, firstly, what adults' reactions were to the young people's sexual knowledges and views on sex education; secondly, what all participants saw as the difficulties, challenges and benefits in integrating the informal and school knowledges of young people; and, thirdly, what participants, especially teachers, thought of the potential of using this data to develop a hybrid curriculum for HIV/AIDS and sexuality education in their local contexts.

Questions for the dialogue

When we had presented the data to the assembled groups, we framed the dialogue around children's sexual knowledges and sex education. We used the following opening questions to begin the discussion:

1. What do you think of the data you have heard and seen? Are you surprised, not surprised, shocked, angered, pleased?
2. Will it make you do anything differently?
3. Do you think we should use young people's knowledge as part of HIV/AIDS and sex education?

If they said yes, then we asked:

4. How do you think it can be used?
5. What are the challenges of using young people's sexual knowledges in school? (We were looking to explore the social, educational and personal challenges.)

After showing a composite video produced in all three countries in the study, which illustrated how students would like sex education to be delivered, we asked the following:

6. What do you notice as the main things that students want?
7. What do you think of the students' views?
8. How is teaching about sex and AIDS different from other teaching for teachers?
9. How do you think we should decide what is in sex and HIV/AIDS education classes and how should it be taught?
10. Should we create an atmosphere or climate in which teachers and students can talk honestly to each other? If so how?
11. What sort of support do schools need to work differently?
12. Are there cultural and religious issues about dealing with sex and HIV/AIDS? How should schools deal with them?

Varying discourses in the dialogues

There were many different discourses evident in the dialogues. Across the three countries there were also variations in the tone, tenor and nature of the dialogues. These differences, although possibly attributable to the way in which dialogues were convened and the levels of participation in each country, also captured the many possible positions that could be adopted towards increasing collaboration in AIDS and sex education. These varying discourses ultimately gave a good representation of the different aspects of the debate around HIV/AIDS and sex education in primary-school classrooms.

Moralising discourse

There was a moralising discourse, which consisted of warning against the dangers of sex education and arguing for the need for all parties (parents, community members, the government, NGOs and religious institutions) to act appropriately. The quotations from teachers in South Africa and Tanzania that follow illustrate this:

> Yes, but the challenge is that home realities are distorted and those realities don't seem to teach them the right moral values. (Unidentified teacher, School B, South Africa)

> I disagree that what has been said by the students is good since from what they see, they have to follow what is good and leave behind what is bad/immoral. How would they know then what is good/moral and what is bad/immoral? Upbringing is how to live according to Almighty's guidance since he has showed us the way of how to live avoiding all this. Therefore we should all change and our children will follow us by abiding by religious scripts in teaching since there is no other way. (Community religion teacher, School A, Tanzania)

In this discourse the adults were often struggling with the role of moral agent and the task of socialising young people into the mores and accepted practices of the culture, as well as the task of keeping them safe from HIV/AIDS and sexual activity. The need to regulate was seen as important, and there was the hope that emphasising the moral aspect, or the 'shoulds', would have an influence. Ms Kidude, a teacher from School A, Tanzania, summarised this view: 'Students should follow the teachings of their parents/guardians/religious leaders/teachers and avoid temptations… Students should avoid imitating bad-mannered children whom were not raised well.'

Children were once again constructed as passive, innocent and likely to be activated by sexual knowledge – as they were in the interviews with teachers and stakeholders described in Chapter 6. In addition, there was frequently a moral element to even discussing sexual matters with children. It was clear that for many it was expected that there should be silence between children and adults on sexual matters.

Educational discourse

There was an educational discourse that acknowledged the special place of the school in the community and the power of the educator to act differently from other adults: 'The school should teach them to endure these challenges they face because you cannot change the environment outside the school but [you can] within the school' (community member, School A, South Africa). The argument was that the school needed to equip learners to not 'just say yes' to the pressures and temptations found outside the school grounds. Children needed to be taught to question what they see at home and in the community, to be more critical and to be decision-makers. In fact, there was agreement in all countries and among all participants that HIV/AIDS-related education was the responsibility of the school and the teacher, and as a result of seeing the pupils' data participants were of the mind that schools should try to engage in open and appropriate education. Ms Kafumu (School B, Tanzania) summarised the consensus: 'HIV/AIDS and sexual education should not be a secret. We should all collaborate across all peer ages'.

There was less agreement about how this should happen, who should take on this role and whether teachers felt prepared and confident to do it. Many teachers wanted others, particularly specialists, to do this. A teacher in School C, Kenya, talked of needing a 'mediator' between the informal and formal knowledge of the pupils. There was a call for a specialist curriculum with professionals from outside of the school responsible for the teaching and learning. Some wanted clear guidelines as to what to teach and what not to teach, with a book that answers learners' questions directly. There was a sense in some of these sections of the dialogue that for some this would be a relief from the complexity, sensitivity and difficulty of the task. However, others relished the idea of engaging more fully and felt that they needed to do that.

Community leadership discourse

There were different views on how the teacher should bridge the clearly visible divide between the community and the school. Some felt that this was a fearful endeavour and that one should tread carefully. Some teachers were scared that parents might 'scold you out' or be accused of 'teaching the child bad manners' by talking to them about sexual matters. Others saw the school as a leader in the community, and the agent of cohesion, an institution that should be educating the community, as described by Ms Kerubo (School C, Kenya) as part of a longer discussion to which we will later return:

Whenever we have school meetings with parents it is very important for somebody to [take a] stand. A teacher [should] talk to parents about sex and HIV/AIDS because we might take it for granted that they know everything and you might find out that some of these things they don't know. So it is very important we educate the parents.

Cultural tension discourse

There was an acknowledgement of the cultural tensions and traditions that made teaching about AIDS and sexuality difficult:

Others will take that you are going against the morals of that community. Traditions and culture are compelling teachers not to speak freely on the issues of HIV/AIDS. Children living in a risk environment can easily understand but those living in good residential areas cannot understand [so] straightforwardly. (Mr Omar, School A, Tanzania)

The challenge that I face is that it is very hard to mention about sexual issues to a child since it is contrary to African customs and traditions. It is also hard because we doubt that by doing so you may be giving that child some knowledge that he or she was not aware of before due to the environment or settings that he or she lives in. (Ms Rose, School A, Tanzania)

Varying locations of power and agency

In addition to the varying discourses in the dialogues, participants also exhibited different positions or expressions of power and agency. Some teachers seemed to see power and agency as very distant from them. For many, it was located in the government and in parents and church leaders. Few conveyed a sense of their own agency. This seemed to be especially pronounced in some of the dialogues. In other dialogues there was a view that teachers, community members and pupils could act together and that consulting and working with pupils was a way of solving the considerable problems raised by AIDS and HIV/AIDS education. Some teachers appeared to be less sure of their position in relation to the surrounding community and openly feared complaining or upset parents. The following comment made by Mr Omar, a teacher from School A, Tanzania, exemplifies this: 'Teachers feel shy when teaching about HIV/AIDS maybe because they have not prepared themselves well or they are frightened of the parents of those students.'

In all the dialogues, there was a consensus that the exercise of consulting pupils was worthwhile; that many had come to understand that young people were sexually aware; and that there was potential in engaging with young people's informal sexual knowledge and views on sex education as a way of enhancing HIV/AIDS education and of engaging with the problems presented by AIDS. Many recognised the authenticity of the photos and comments of the pupils, and the adults recognised the social worlds reflected in them:

> We are faced by the challenge of looking for different ways through which we can deliver the message to these children to prevent them from falling into temptations. We should educate the society so that they understand that their children are not too young and that they know about issues of sexual intercourse. (Mr Twaha, School A, Tanzania)

However, there was also an acknowledgement that the dialogue was an unusual event and one that needed support and outside facilitation. In Kenya, the actors were especially enthusiastic about the activity, as evidenced by Ms Kerubo's enthusiastic thank you to the facilitator at the end of the dialogue:

> [Speaking to the researcher] You are an asset to us [clapping]. I hope this is not the last forum that we have with you and the other stakeholders…we are so grateful…We are grateful having somebody like you with us…this forum has helped us. I would like to have you every now and then [clapping].

The possibility of change

There was one passage of dialogue that exemplified the nature of dialogue, its capacity and its potential to bring about a different form of discourse. In the rather lengthy passage that follows, the engagement in an unusually open form of dialogue is apparent and the shifts of understanding are evident. It contains the qualities Burbules (1993) describes: respect and equality among the actors; reaching a shared and different understanding that builds on what is already known; and a clear, almost disciplined, focus.

In this section of dialogue, the group in Kenya respond to a boy pupil who asked what they would do if a young person told them he has had sex. They discuss how there is a need to educate, but also to be appropriate.

Grandmother: When a child says that he or she is used to having sex, this is as a result of mistakes we parents have made where our children are concerned. For example, a parent chooses to sleep in the same room with their 12-year-old son or daughter. Therefore the activities that take place between you and the man, our children are seeing far and wide whatever you are doing. That child is not sleeping. The child watches and sees what is my mother doing. Such a child starts practising the same thing he or she has been watching. The duty of us parents is to protect our children even though we are poor. We should not wait when a child is 12 years to give them a room of their own, because at times when a child is just three years old, you find that such a child can be watching what takes place between the father and mother and starts practising that subject. Therefore we parents should take that responsibility, placing our children in other rooms so that they do not see that activity. Thank you.

Female chief:	It has already been agreed that we should start teaching our children sex education at an early age. Mine is still on the language issue [the terminology to be used for speaking about sex]. Mama C…has already said that we tell them '*jongo*' [a euphemism for 'penis', used instead of 'mboro']. [Laughter] When we tell them *jongo* they will continue using the word *jongo*. I would like this forum to be used to decide the language that should be used. Like in standard 1 do I tell them the exact word or…?
Many:	Yes!
Ms Kerubo:	What do I do? Or do I use the language we use like when we were being taught science, in standard 7 or in standard 8 or do we use *jongo* instead of telling them *mtoto analetwa na ndege* [children are brought by aeroplanes]. May I know that one?
Many:	[Group express surprise and laughter.]
Ms Kerubo:	Shh! [asks for quiet]. Okay, I think in the school the teacher – whenever we have school meetings with parents – it is very important for somebody to [take a] stand. A teacher to talk to parents about sex and HIV/AIDS because we might take it for granted that they know everything and you might find out that some of these things they don't know. So it is very important we educate the parents. And also when we are in school, during our discussions with our pupils – let us bring them close to us so that they are free to ask any questions they want.
Kustiantu (boy):	If a lady is a virgin or another can no longer have children, and they have sex with someone who has AIDS, will these two ladies get AIDS? [Laughter then silence and murmurs in the audience.]
Mr Mbogo:	First of all, I did not understand the question. Did he ask that when someone who is a virgin and has sex with someone who has HIV/AIDS, can he get HIV/AIDS?
Researcher:	Yes.
Mr Mbogo:	Yes he can get HIV/AIDS. Even if she's a virgin or not.
Ms Ngina:	She has done sex with someone who has AIDS.
Mr Mbogo:	Yes she did sex with someone who has HIV/AIDS. So she can get HIV/AIDS even if she's a virgin. Whether you have stopped giving birth, whether you are a virgin, and you have sex with an HIV-positive man, you will be infected. Why? Because what transmits the infection, is the liquid. Men produce semen and women also have a juice in the body, so the exchange of the liquids, which is found in either virgins or women who have stopped giving birth, the liquid is still found in both. So once there is exchange of liquid, then you get infected.
Researcher:	Yes.
Mr Mbogo:	Have I answered you? So it is the liquid and not the state of the lady at that particular time that is a factor. Okay?

This dialogue illustrates a number of phenomena. Here we see the gradual seriousness of tone developing and the reaction to the boy who seizes the opportunity to ask a question about sex and HIV/AIDS. He seems to feel safe here to engage with the adults in a different way. The two older women lead a very deep reflection on the question and the rest of the group are drawn into treating this dialogue as meaningful and demanding a different attitude and language. The stigmas and embarrassments are overcome and serious interaction between adults and children on a very serious topic is modelled. This, in turn, leads to yet another serious question being asked of the group by Kustiantu – with similar results.

The question this dialogue raises is whether this can be recreated in a classroom. Can this environment and this process help teachers and pupils engage in the very complex sociocultural task of discussing honestly matters of sex and HIV/AIDS? Is it possible to do so within the contexts of community and parental fears and taboos?

The power of stories and of drawing on the reality of the lives of the actors in this dialogue is also apparent. This is of course something that the children also asked for in their consultation. They wanted to use stories and role plays to learn. They recognised narrative as a way of engaging with the reality of their lives, but by focusing on the story and the characters, it was less threatening and personally exposing.

Our experience of dialogues in all three countries does suggest that there is potential in such processes for adults and young people to interact in complex and sensitive topics in a culture that has emphasised silence on these matters.

CHAPTER 8

Improving practice and effecting change

In this book we have offered important perspectives on the need to talk to children about sex education, especially in an age of HIV/AIDS. We have taken seriously those scholars who advocate consulting pupils, including sociologist Ann Oakley (1994: 25), who asks: 'What would it really mean to study the world from the standpoint of children both as knowers and as actors?' In Chapter 1 we noted that two-thirds of all HIV infections in the world are to be found in sub-Saharan Africa. We also spoke of education as the social vaccine against HIV infection in the absence of a medical cure. Since HIV is primarily sexually transmitted, the pandemic has caused parents, teachers and community workers to reconsider the issue of sex education for children and young people. Young people's risk of HIV infection is heightened in sub-Saharan Africa because of high levels of poverty and low levels of education. This makes effective sex education an even more pressing need. However, given the cultural and religious values operating in these African communities, as well as the cultural understanding of knowledge and the existing relationships between children and adults, sex education is no easy task.

Even without the spectre of AIDS and the influence of culture, sex education has always been a contested arena. Some have argued vehemently that exposure leads to experimentation, whereas others have asserted that knowledge equips young people, empowering them to make informed decisions. Alongside these two views, there is a perspective that advocates strongly for maintaining children's innocence for as long as possible. Yet others, including this study, provide evidence for children's extant and vigilant awareness of a highly sexualised world – and argue that children are at risk if treated as innocents. The data we have collected over the course of two years in Tanzania, Kenya and South Africa suggest that the answers to how we deal with children and sex education lie somewhere between innocence and exposure, and somewhere beyond the usual features of cultural impediments to learning. Before we discuss these, we briefly summarise the findings of our study.

A summary of findings

On young people's sexual knowledges we found that children have wide-ranging and fairly sophisticated knowledge of adults' sexual practices and sexual worlds, such as prostitution, the influence of drugs and alcohol, and rape and prostitution. They observe sexual acts regularly and are well aware of the particular practices in their environs. The young people were primary-aged pupils in this study, so we can assume that this awareness is formulated at a fairly young age. They understand well the consequences of unprotected sex and HIV/AIDS and are keen to avoid them. They want a lot more information and dialogue with adults on sexual matters and HIV/AIDS in particular. Furthermore, they are aware that they cannot share this knowledge with adults. Indeed, adults are often ambivalent and avoid talking to young people honestly and openly about sexual matters and HIV/AIDS.

On sex education in schools, we found that children want a more interactive and active pedagogy that allows them to engage with their own knowledge and to talk about their lack of knowledge. They are concerned that the information they get is unrealistic and does not reflect the world in which they live. Teachers affirmed what pupils said about current HIV/AIDS education – though there were a few who tried to be open about sexuality. Teachers want to help, but not many are confident or feel well resourced. Teachers articulated numerous challenges to their practice, mostly identifying technical and social issues that impede their complete participation in HIV/AIDS-education delivery. Some are more frightened of engaging in discussions about HIV/AIDS than others. There is a fear in particular of disapproval from parents and community leaders. The school or the practices in school are influenced by the wider community and the dominant attitudes of the community (e.g. religion and cultural practices). Therefore, the school is a mirror of the community in which it is located. There are very different conceptions about the values and approaches that might be effective and which of these should be adopted.

In a later phase of our study, we held dialogues among all three groups of our study participants – children, teachers and community stakeholders. Our theory of change was that the way to shift attitudes and engage with the sexual knowledge of young people might be to share the findings of the data on young people's sexual knowledge and their preferred form of sex education. When we did this, we found that adults (teachers, parents and community leaders) were surprised at and interested in the extent and nature of the young people's knowledge. Community stakeholders, though supportive of HIV/AIDS education in the school, felt that it should be taught within the confines of a protective discourse. Nevertheless, adults were generally willing to engage with the idea of non-naïve young people and that this fact offered a different possibility in terms of sex and HIV/AIDS education. Adults seemed open to the potential for dialogue about HIV/AIDS education for their young people, although some intractable problems remained.

In reflecting on our findings and thinking ahead to how they might influence practice, we have located two important learnings regarding innocence and culture, and their relation to the sex and AIDS education curriculum in school, which we will address in turn.

Between innocence and exposure/empowerment

In all our primary schools, in all three country sites, we observed indications of children's exposure to sexualised behaviour and sexual activity. Their home and community environments have exposed them to 'live sex'. Children bring these sexual knowledges from home and the community into school – although they frequently leave it at the door of the classroom. The secret sexual lives they know about and live are seldom discussed in the classroom. Instead, they and the adults in their lives (including their teachers) enact an elaborate charade of 'the innocence of childhood' along with a structured and organised way of learning. These public sexual lives that children see and from which they derive everyday knowledge are in sharp contrast to the formal curriculum taught in school. The insulation and boundary between the two is strong and clear. The school context offers factual information and prohibitive and protective discourse which is removed from the pupils' lived experiences. Meanwhile, everyday knowledges provide unfiltered information, from which children could benefit through discussion. In fact, throughout our study children made it clear that they want to make sense of what they see through discussion with trusted adults. Teachers, especially, are the ones with whom they wish to engage and we can hypothesise that this is because of the particular role and relationship teachers have with children, especially in the primary age group. Teachers are seen as being different to parents, especially with regard to education in the sexual domain.

Our data have shown children having a knowledgeable and sophisticated sexual world both in and out of the school – one which they are fully capable of articulating. A protective and repressive discourse does not seem appropriate for these young people. They know about sexual encounters: they see such encounters in buses, bushes, brothels, cemeteries and *keshas*. Some are engaged in sexual activity themselves. Their voices captured in our study show that they would want teachers (and other adults) to engage with these experiences in a comprehensive and interactive way. Arguably, pupils trust their teachers and want to be able to confide in them. How do teachers and parents respond to these implicit and overt requests for change to the way things have always been done?

Joanne Faulkner (2011) talks of how protecting childhood innocence enables adults to keep their own feelings of alienation and powerlessness at bay. It is a way of dealing with our own identity and fears about the world in which we live, together with its dangers and disappointments. As a result, there is an overvaluation of innocence; it is leading to an increasingly secluded and sentimentalised view of the importance of maintaining children as innocent. Faulkner's (2011: 68) analysis draws on philosophical and religious notions in which 'children are prone to impiety and in need of firm authority'. Key to her solution is the need for children to be seen as agents and citizens who can be involved in 'a deliberative, democratic practice' (Faulkner 2011: 76). She further argues that '[c]hildren are as capable as adults of responding to others' views if such views are offered in the spirit of reciprocity' (Faulkner 2011: 76). This we saw in the dialogues as well as in the various other techniques we used in order to elicit children's view on sex education and to interrogate their sexual knowledges.

Perhaps most powerfully, Faulkner (2011: 76) argues that 'involvement in family and community decision making not only empowers children, but also allows them to experience…responsibility…agency and freedom'. This she believes to be a practice 'more rewarding than exercising authority over children and underestimating their capacities…[and makes adults]… less prone to indulge projective fantasies of savages, not quite humans, and innocents in need of protection' (Faulkner 2011: 77). Though speaking in the context of families, Faulkner's vision may easily be extended to a school context. It does mean, however, that more consultation is required in order to ensure that parents and teachers are working towards a common goal and that teachers are not afraid to teach in the way that best serves the interests and needs of children.

Faulkner (2011: 128) concludes by arguing that:

> Teenage desire and our inability to control it heightens adults' sense of vulnerability and helplessness and signals a loss of the sweet refuge from worry and work that childhood innocence is supposed to represent. To move beyond fear and towards more productive ways of coping with adolescents' passage from childhood to adulthood would require an attention to the views of children that is not yet evident in our culture.

In writing from Western perspectives and for Western families, Faulkner's views capture those of the adults in our study. To be sure, parents, teachers and community leaders we encountered displayed varying senses of the helplessness that Faulkner describes. She advocates 'relinquishing our investment in the idea of childhood innocence understood in terms of ignorance and protection' (Faulkner 2011: 126) in order to better serve children through open discussion that will ultimately protect them to a far greater extent than keeping them ignorant or innocent in a world that is far from it.

Of course, it may be argued that different communities have different needs regarding childhood innocence. For example, does the same argument apply in a middle-class community where children are not as exposed to 'live sex' as the young people in our study were? Is there not an argument to be made for protecting children until close to the time when they may need the information, rather than unnecessarily burdening them too soon? These are not easy questions to answer, but need to be interrogated in the context of community norms and experiences. Furthermore, in our study we have not differentiated between children who may be extremely protected and naïve and those who are not. Nor have we measured the range of explicit everyday knowledges within a class. It is our analysis that the social context of the community in which the school is located – and from which the children originate – means that children's everyday knowledges are similar. Though we have not tested this assumption empirically, our observations would support such a conclusion.

Everyday knowledges are likely to differ between communities and within a community. Even children who are protected by parents and religious and cultural practices observe the realities in their midst. And irrespective of the environment, these 'open discussions' still come up against cultural impediments. But perhaps these are not as insurmountable as they may first seem.

Beyond cultural impediments to learning

In the course of both our primary and secondary research, we repeatedly encountered teachers' lack of preparation and confidence in teaching sex and HIV/AIDS education in sub-Saharan Africa. For many, the controlling and lecture-led discourses and patterns of interaction seem to arise both from a lack of technical skills (theory, reflection on practice and preparation) and from cultural impediments to learning.

In much of this study we captured the voices of parents, teachers and children as they explained at length, and in some detail, the cultural obstacles to teaching and learning about sex education. Children mentioned how adults rarely spoke of sex, though they were frequently exposed to it in their homes and communities, as well as through media. Grandparents reiterated the cultural taboos in which parents did not speak to children, although there were some adults, such as initiation school teachers, aunts and older siblings, who were mandated to do so (Van der Heijden & Swartz 2010).

These observations also connect to the position adopted by the school in relation to the community, especially with regard to sex and HIV/AIDS education. Again, we saw different positions being adopted. In some cases, the schools perceived their role to be that of change agents leading the way in giving a widely conceived education on HIV/AIDS. In other cases, schools saw themselves as reflections of community attitudes and were fearful of challenging the status quo. In moving beyond these cultural impediments to learning, we must now seek to answer the questions, what sort of support would teachers need to engage in effective, interactive HIV/AIDS education? And what can aid teachers in the perceived clash of expectations between their community and their classroom?

In writing on the relationship between pedagogy and culture, Robin Alexander (1999, 2000) offers a non-ethnocentric way of viewing both questions when he states that 'teaching is an act while pedagogy is both act and discourse...Pedagogy connects the apparently self-contained act of teaching with culture, structure and mechanisms of social control' (Alexander 2000: 540). He highlights a trio of key factors – knowledge, the learner and the teacher – in the relationship between culture and pedagogy. In our study we have learnt a great deal about all three of these, the multiple ways in which they are rooted in culture and the tensions that exist between them.

With regard to knowledge, we have seen first-hand the reliance on formal, factual knowledge and the use of the book as the authoritative source. Teachers told us and showed us the importance of providing an authoritative response. They did so for two reasons – to protect themselves from criticism and because this is the cultural model with which they grew up. There is an overwhelming expectation that they will be transmitters of factual and definitive information. The Bernsteinian framework that helped us distinguish vertical from horizontal and everyday from formal was enormously useful in this regard (and will be returned to later).

As for teachers, we have seen their dilemmas very clearly, especially with respect to their preparation and teaching. You cannot teach what you are not confident to teach. And you cannot vary your pedagogy if it is the only transmission model with which you are familiar. Teachers – their selection, preparation and ability – are key to education; in the contexts in which we researched it was clear to see the complexity of their positions and the sociocultural tug of war in which they find themselves. Teachers see and feel the immediate pressures and needs of the pupils – we have evidence of that. But we also see teachers caught up in the silences, stigmas and preconceptions of their culture. They have not been prepared to engage pedagogically in the sort of interaction and learning that the pupils want, namely answering real questions about real-life dilemmas. As a result, they lack confidence and choose not to engage. This suggests that a different sort of training and preparation is needed for teachers in order to equip them adequately to provide sex and AIDS education. Most importantly, consensus through consultation with stakeholders is essential in order for teachers to be given permission to pursue a different kind of education.

With regard to the learner, teachers have a choice to make regarding whether to keep them passive recipients or view them as sexual actors and inhabitants of a complex sexual world. From our data it is clear that children desire to engage in schooling and classroom practice. They showed us the very complex situations with which matters of HIV and sexuality presented them. They also displayed both agency and interpretive ability in making sense of these. Their judgements routinely navigate life-and-death situations. They want to bring these processes, situations and discussions (i.e. their informal knowledge) into school and they have clearly told us that they see teachers as the adults who can inform them and help them engage with this complex world. They want a more dialogic form of pedagogy. They are asking for a hybrid curriculum and for help in negotiating complexity. The adults know about the context to some extent, but are ambivalent and caught in the authoritative transmission model of knowledge that is their cultural and historical model. In our study we have seen that, even in impoverished contexts, children and adults are able to change the status quo, though the inertia to do so is great and sometimes overwhelming.

Finally, Alexander (2000: 27) suggests that opportunities for change to pedagogy and the curriculum are 'vastly increased and enriched if we extend it beyond the boundaries of one school to others, one region to others, one culture to others and one country to others'. The challenges that children and teachers face in the three countries in which we conducted our fieldwork are not unique. In all societies religious, cultural and moral mores are frequently at odds with progressive learner-centred approaches. Innocence is valued all over the world; adulthood is associated with authority. Consultation is necessarily time-consuming and fraught, but demands reflection on practice. Jacob (2009: 313) calls for 'reflective HIV education design' and describes this reflective practice as 'a balancing act':

> Reflective HIV and AIDS education design is an ongoing balancing act; it requires participation by all key stakeholders who have the necessary ownership to achieve a unified goal…Reflective designers of programmes must balance or address many elements. These include culture, religion, access to information and technology, costs, and relevance to local, national, regional, and international contexts.

Both Alexander and Jacob's analyses are essential for changing pedagogy. In concluding this study, we return to Basil Bernstein and the many ways in which he has provided us with analytical lenses and action steps towards changing the way in which sex and AIDS education is approached with children.

Back to Bernstein and consulting pupils

Throughout this study we have used Bernstein's insights to guide our understandings and interpretations of data. We began with a material interest in understanding how everyday knowledges interacted with formal knowledges. We discovered that with regard to sex and HIV/AIDS education, they seldom did. In Chapter 6 we spoke of 'weakly framed' curricula with regard to the content of sex and AIDS education. For Bernstein, 'framing' is related to the transmission of knowledge through pedagogic practices. Framing refers to where the control lies when communication takes place in a classroom, and 'the degree of control teacher and pupil possess over the selection, organization, pacing and timing of the knowledge transmitted and received in the pedagogical relationship' (Bernstein 1973: 88). According to Bernstein (1990b: 100), 'framing regulates the form of its legitimate message'. Strong framing, therefore, refers to a limited degree of options for the teacher and students; weak framing implies more freedom. It seems appropriate for sex and AIDS education to be weakly framed. It also allows for the incorporation of everyday knowledge into the formal school curriculum.

Another of Bernstein's ideas of relevance here is his distinction between a competence and performance curriculum. In a competence curriculum Bernstein (1996) asserts that the aim is to develop learners' innate competencies. Competence curricula are characterised by integration between subjects and strong links are made between school learning and real life. Knowledge is not imposed from outside, but is instead drawn out and is based on learners' own experiences and everyday knowledge. This focus on learners' own experiences builds confidence. In the context of the skills needed to navigate life in a sexualised world not always safe for children, this confidence is an important contribution to protecting children. This is another way in which children can be protected, and, notably one that does not result in shielding them from important discussions about information they already have. In this respect, protection is not from innocence but from harm. For Bernstein, like Freire, a competence curriculum is concerned with education as an act of emancipation – building competence in children's lives in order to assist them in overcoming their social contexts and situations. The role of a teacher in a competence curriculum is as the facilitator of learning. This is especially important in order to address the fear that teachers face in teaching knowledge that is deemed inappropriate or culturally frowned upon.

Conclusion

In this study we have offered detailed data about the nature, sources and processes of the knowledges that young people bring into the classroom. We have begun to understand how children acquire their knowledge, what importance is attached to different sources, the ways in which poverty produces specific knowledges and how these knowledges interact with existing curricula and pedagogies. In the main, children know a lot about sex, but are forced to hide this knowledge in the more formal spaces of classroom and home. The most interesting finding is that while children are not keen to experiment with this knowledge, they are curious: what happens if condoms break? How do gay people have sex? How does the virus work?

Throughout, we have argued for a more 'open-ended' pedagogy in which teaching practices are 'participatory, more interactive, adventurous, learner-centred' (Dembélé & Lefoka 2007: 536). We noted that such practices are challenging in sub-Saharan African classrooms not only because of the barriers of inadequate resources and training, but also because of the incongruence between these pedagogies and teachers' views on the nature of knowledge, the purpose of education and the desired relationships between adults and children.

In the course of the two years in which we have sought to consult pupils, teachers and stakeholders, possibly our most important conclusion concerns what happens when these three groups of actors are placed in dialogue with each other. Although all three groups initially repeated their fears and concerns, it became apparent that given enough time and space a new pedagogy and new curricula might be possible.

In all dialogues there was growing consensus that the exercise of consulting pupils was worthwhile. Parents, religious leaders and teachers came to understand that children were sexually aware, but not precocious. Children had to cope and engage with their lived realities and make sense of them, and choose to act in context. They were not waiting for opportunities to experiment, but to talk, discuss and negotiate. They were curious about mechanics and details, opportunities for activism and the experiences of others.

As the dialogues progressed so too did a gradual seriousness of tone. Children, often silent for long periods during the dialogues, grew in confidence as the discussion progressed, and were encouraged to ask questions and participate with adults in a different way. Reflections and questions deepened as the groups began treating this dialogue as meaningful. All participants began to recognise that such an engagement demanded a different attitude and language. Stigmas and embarrassments were addressed and serious interaction between adults and children was modelled.

So we have evidence that suggests these consultations and dialogues can help teachers and pupils engage in the complex sociocultural task of discussing honestly matters of sex and HIV/AIDS. However, a more important question remains unanswered. Is it possible for these dialogues to be recreated in African classrooms in urban and rural areas? During dialogues there was a frank acknowledgement that the meeting was an unusual event and one that needed support and outside facilitation. This was especially critical within the contexts of community and parental fears, taboos and silence.

Based on our data and experiences in both the consultations and dialogues, we are impelled to advocate a weakly framed sex- and AIDS-education curriculum. We see in our data the working models of practice for both schools and classrooms that take seriously the challenges for teachers, pupils and policy-makers. For children, we have seen the complexity of their knowledge and the silence between them and the adults.

We have seen the ways in which adults attempt to perpetuate the myth that young people do not (or ought not to) know anything about the sexual aspects of life. At the same time, we have seen the possibility for adults to be dissuaded of this viewpoint when confronted with evidence to the contrary. We have also shown the sophistication of children's thinking in regard to their lived realities and their desire to be helped to understand what is going on around them. They want a 'hybrid' curriculum – one that is led by teachers but informed by their own experiences. Finally, we have seen very clearly, how schools are uniquely placed as bridges between home, community culture and children. They offer a pathway through the complexity of taboos and fear.

These consultations and dialogues offer a powerful possibility for change and a new form of pedagogy and curriculum. The work for the future very much lies in how to achieve this in a way that is replicable and sustainable.

References

Acedo C (2009) Editorial. *Prospects* 39(4): 307–309

Ackers J & Hardman F (2001) Classroom interaction in Kenyan primary schools. *Compare* 31(2): 245–261

Aggleton P & Campbell C (2000) Working with young people – Towards an agenda for sexual health. *Sexual & Relationship Therapy* 15(3): 283–296

Aggleton P & Crewe M (2005) Editorial: Effects and effectiveness in sex and relationships education. *Sex Education*, 5(4): 303–306

Ahlberg BM & Pertet AM (2006) A map of the complexities that have emerged in HIV and AIDS research. In A Pertet (Ed.) *Re-thinking research and intervention approaches that aim at preventing HIV infection among the youth*. Nairobi: The Regal Press Kenya Ltd.

Aikman S, Unterhalter E & Boler T (2008) *Gender equality, HIV, and AIDS. A challenge for the education sector*. Oxford: Oxfam

Airhihenbuwa C & Obregon R (2000) A critical assessment of theories/models used in health communication for HIV/AIDS. *Journal of Health Communication* 5: 5–15

Alexander R (1999) Culture in pedagogy, pedagogy across cultures. In R Alexander, P Broadfoot & D Phillips (Eds) *Learning from comparing: New directions in comparative education research*, vol.1: 149–180. Oxford: Symposium Books

Alexander R (2000) *Culture and pedagogy: International comparisons in primary education*. Oxford: Blackwell

Al-Hinai AM (2007) The interplay between culture, teacher professionalism and teachers' professional development at times of change. In T Townsend & R Bates (Eds) *Handbook of teacher education*. Netherlands: Springer

Allen L (2005) *Sexual subjects: Young people, sexuality and education*. London: Palgrave Macmillan

Allen L (2007) Denying the sexual subject: Schools' regulation of student sexuality. *British Educational Research Journal* 33(2): 221–234

Altinyelken HK (2010) Pedagogical renewal in sub-Saharan Africa: The case of Uganda. *Comparative Education* 46(2): 151–171

Arnot M, McIntyre D, Pedder D & Reay D (2004) *Consultation in the classroom: Developing dialogue about teaching and learning*. Cambridge: Pearson Publishing

Aved B & Zones J (1985) Promoting parental involvement in sex education in California. *American Journal of Public Health* 75(5): 563–564

Baker DP, Collins JM & Leon J (2009) Risk factor or social vaccine? The historical progression of the role of education in HIV and AIDS infection in sub-Saharan Africa. *Prospects* 38 (4): 467–486

Banyard K (2010) The equality illusion. London: Faber and Faber

Bedi A, Kimalu P, Manda D & Nafula N (2002) *The decline in primary enrolment in Kenya*. Nairobi: Kenya Institute for Policy Research and Analysis

Bennell PS, Hyde K & Swainson N (2002) *The impact of the HIV/AIDS epidemic on the education sector in sub-Saharan Africa: A synthesis of the findings and recommendations of three country studies*. Brighton, UK: Sussex University

Bernstein B (1971) On the classification and framing of educational knowledge. In M Young (Ed.) *Knowledge and control: New directions for the sociology of education*. London: Macmillan

Bernstein B (1973) *Class, codes and control*, vol. 2. London: Routledge & Kegan Paul

Bernstein B (1990a) *The structuring of pedagogic discourse*. London: Routledge

Bernstein B (1990b) *Class, codes and control, vol. 4: The structuring of pedagogic discourse*. London: Routledge

Bernstein B (1996) *Pedagogy, symbolic control, and identity: Theory, research, critique*. London: Taylor & Francis

Bernstein B (1999) Vertical and horizontal discourse: An essay. *British Journal of Sociology of Education* 20(2): 157–173

Bettinghaus P (1986) Health promotion and the knowledge-attitude-behavior continuum. *Preventive Medicine* 15(5): 475–491

Bhana D (2007a) Beyond stigma: Young children's responses to HIV and AIDS. *Culture, Health and Sexuality* 10(7): 725–738

Bhana D (2007b) Childhood sexuality and rights in the context of HIV/AIDS. *Culture, Health & Sexuality* 9(3): 309–324

Bhana D (2007c) The price of innocence: Teachers, gender, childhood sexuality, HIV and AIDS in early schooling. *International Journal of Inclusive Education*, 11(4): 431–444

Blake S (2002) *Sex and relationship education: A step-by-step guide for teachers*. London: David Fulton Publishers

Boler T & Aggleton R (2004) *HIV/AIDS and education. Life skills-based education for HIV prevention: A critical analysis*. London: Save the Children and ActionAid International

Boler T & Aggleton P (2005) *Life skills-based education for HIV prevention: A critical analysis*. London: Save the Children and ActionAid International

Bourdieu P (1989) Social space and symbolic power. *Sociological Theory* 7(1): 14–25

Bragg S (2007) 'Student Voice' and governmentality: The production of enterprising subjects? *Discourse: Studies in the Cultural Politics of Education* 28(3): 343–358

Bridges D (1988) *Education, democracy and discussion*. Slough: NFER/Nelson

Brown AD, Jejeebhoy SJ, Shah I & Yount KM (2001) *Sexual relations among young people in developing countries: Evidence from WHO case studies*. Geneva: Department of Reproductive Health and Research, World Health Organization

Bryk F (1933) *Voodoo-EROS: Ethnological studies in the sex-life of the African aborigines*. New York: Syd Sculdiner

Bunyi G (1997) Multi-lingualism and discourse in primary mathematics in Kenya. *Culture and Curriculum* 10(1): 23–30

Burbules NC (1993) *Dialogue in teaching: Theory and practice*. New York: Teachers College Press

Burbules NC & Hansen DT (Eds) (1997) *Teaching and its predicaments*. Oxford: Westview Press

Campbell C (2003) *'Letting them die': Why HIV/AIDS prevention programmes fail*. Indiana University Press

Campbell C, Foulis CA, Maiman S & Sibiya Z (2005) The impact of social environments on the effectiveness of youth HIV prevention: A South African case study. *AIDS Care* 17(4): 471–478

Campbell C & MacPhail C (2002) Peer education, gender and the development of critical consciousness: Participatory HIV prevention by South African young people. *Social Science & Medicine* 55(2): 331–345

Central Intelligence Agency (2010) *The world fact book – Kenya*, https://www.cia.gov/library/publications/the-world-factbook/geos/ke.html

Chege F & Sifuna D (2006) *Girls' and women's education in Kenya: Gender perspectives and trends*. Nairobi: UNESCO

Chick JK (1996) Safe-talk, collusion in apartheid education. In H Coleman (Ed.) *Society and the language classroom*. Cambridge: Cambridge University Press

Chisholm L & Leyendecker R (2008) Curriculum reform in post-1990s sub-Saharan Africa. *International Journal of Educational Development* 28(2): 195–205

Coleman J (2010) *The nature of adolescence* (4th edition). London: Routledge

Cooley CH (1967) *Human nature and social order*. New York: Shocken Books

Coombe C & Kelly MJ (2002) *Education as a vehicle for combating HIV/AIDS*. Paris: UNESCO

Davidson E (2005) Understanding and improving quality in Tanzanian primary schooling. PhD thesis, School of Development Studies, University of East Anglia

Dembélé M & Lefoka P (2007) Pedagogical renewal for quality universal primary education: Overview of trends in sub-Saharan Africa. *International Review of Education* 53(5/6): 531–553

De Waal A (2002) HIV/AIDS and young Africans. In A De Waal & N Argenti (Eds) *Young Africa: Realising the rights of children and youth*. Trenton, NJ and Asmara: Africa World Press Inc.

DoE (South Africa Department of Education) (1999) *National policy on HIV/Aids, for learners and educators in public schools, and students and educators in further education and training: Institutions* (Government Notice No. 20372). Pretoria: DoE

DoE (2000a) *The HIV and AIDS emergency: Guidelines for educators*. Pretoria: DoE

DoE (2000b) *Norms and standards for educators* (Government Gazette No. 20844). Pretoria: DoE

DoE (2002a) *National curriculum statement grades R–9 life orientation*. Pretoria: DoE

DoE (2002b) *Protecting the right to innocence: The importance of sexuality education.* Pretoria: DoE

DoE (2002c) *Revised national curriculum statement grades R–9 (schools).* Pretoria: DoE

DoE (2009) *Education statistics in South Africa 2008*. Pretoria: DoE

Eastern Africa Network of HIV/AIDS & Education in Eastern Africa (2010), http://www.schoolsandhealth.org/sites/eastafrica/Pages/Kenya.aspx

Elimu Yetu Coalition (2005) The challenge of educating girls in Kenya. In S Aikman & E Unterhalter (Eds) *Beyond access: Transforming policy and practice for gender equality in education.* Oxford, UK: Oxfam

Esat F (2003) *The social construction of 'sexual knowledge': Exploring the narratives of southern African youth of Indian descent in the context of HIV/AIDS.* Master's thesis, Rhodes University, South Africa

Everatt D (1994) *Creating a future: Youth policy for South Africa.* Johannesburg: Ravan Press

Faulkner J (2011) *The importance of being innocent: Why we worry about children.* Cambridge: Cambridge University Press

Festinger L (1957) *A theory of cognitive dissonance.* Stanford, CA, USA: Stanford University Press

Fine M (1988) Sexuality, schooling, and adolescent females: The missing discourse of desire. *Harvard Educational Review* 58(1): 29–53

Flanders NA (1970) *Analyzing teacher behavior.* Reading, Massachusets: Addison-Wesley

Flutter J & Rudduck J (2004) *Consulting pupils: What's in it for schools?* London: Routledge Falmer

Foucault M (1976) *The will to knowledge: The history of sexuality,* vol.1. London: Penguin

Francis D (2010) Sexuality education in South Africa: Three essential questions. *International Journal of Educational Development* 30(3): 314–319

Freire P (1970) *Pedagogy of the oppressed.* New York: Seabury

Freire P (1985) *The politics of education: Culture, power and liberation.* London: Palgrave Macmillan

Gouws E, Stanecki KA, Lyerla R & Ghys PD (2008) The epidemiology of HIV infection among young people aged 15–24 years in southern Africa. AIDS 22(4): 5–16

Gregson S, Waddell H & Chandiwana S (2001) School education and HIV control in sub-Saharan Africa: From harmony to discord. *Journal of International Development* 13: 467–485

Griffiths C, French R, Patel-Kanwal H & Rait G (2008) 'Always between two cultures': Young British Bangladeshis and their mothers' views on sex and relationships. *Culture, Health & Sexuality* 10(7): 709–723

Gupta GR, Parkhurst JO, Ogden JA, Aggleton P & Mahal A (2008) Structural approaches to HIV prevention. *The Lancet* 372: 764–775

Handwerker WP (2001) *Quick ethnography.* Walnut Creek, CA: AltaMira Press

Hardman F, Abd-Kadir J, & Smith F (2008) Pedagogical renewal: Improving the quality of classroom interaction in Nigerian primary schools. *International Journal of Educational Development* 28(4): 955–969

Helleve A, Flisher AJ, Onya H, Kaaya S, Mukoma W et al. (2009a) Teachers' confidence in teaching HIV/AIDS and sexuality in South African and Tanzanian schools. *Scandinavian Journal of Public Health* 37 (Supp. 2): 55–64

Helleve A, Flisher A, Onya H, Mukoma W & Klepp K (2009b) South African teachers' reflections on the impact of culture on their teaching of sexuality and HIV/AIDS. *Cult Health Sex* 11(2):189–204

Hunt F (2009) *Dropping out from school* (CREATE Policy Brief No. 8), http://www.create-rpc.org/pdf_documents/Policy_Brief_8.pdf

Ingham R (2005) 'We didn't cover that at school': Education against pleasure or education for pleasure? *Sex Education* 5(4): 375–388

Jacob WJ (2009) Reflective HIV education design: Balancing current needs with best practice. *Prospects* 39(4): 311–319

Jayahrajah C & Branson W (1993) *Structural and sectoral adjustment: World Bank experience, 1980–1992.* Washington, DC: World Bank

Jeater D (1993) *Marriage, perversion and power: The construction of moral discourse in southern Rhodesia 1894–1930.* Oxford: Clarendon Press

Jewkes R, Martin L & Penn-Kekana L (2002) The virgin cleansing myth: Cases of child rape are not exotic. *The Lancet* (British edition) 359(9307): 711

Jewkes R, Penn-Kekana L, Rose-Junius, H (2005) "If they rape me, I can't blame them": Reflections on gender in the social context of child rape in South Africa and Namibia. *Social Science & Medicine* 61: 1809–1820

Jones M (2004) The effect of participation in the neighbourhood academic program on the auto-photographic self-concepts of inner-city adolescents. *Journal of Instructional Psychology* 31(3): 188–201

KANCO (Kenya AIDS NGOs Consortium) (2008) KANCO *Background*, http://www.kanco.org/FW266/html/moreper cent20infor.html

Kehily MJ (2002) *Sexuality, gender and schooling: Shifting agendas in social learning*. London: Routledge Falmer

Kelly MJ (2000) *The encounter between HIV/AIDS and education*. Harare: UNESCO Sub-Regional Office for Southern Africa

Kenya Demographic and Health Survey (2003) *Kenya Demographic and Health Survey*. Nairobi: Bureau of Statistics

Kenyatta J (1938) *Facing Mount Kenya*. London: Secker & Warburg

Kiragu SW (2007) Exploring sexuality education and the burdened teacher: A participatory approach in a rural primary school in Kenya. *Pastoral Care in Education* 25(3): 5–15

Kiragu SW (2009) *Exploring young people's sexuality in a poor community in Kenya: A case study*. Doctoral thesis, University of Cambridge.

Kirby D (2002) HIV transmission and prevention in adolescents. In L Peiperl & P Volverding (Eds) *HIV InSite Knowledge Base*. San Francisco: University of California

Kirby D (2008) *A history of Uganda's campaign to decrease HIV prevalence in the early 1990s*. California: ETR Associates

Kirby D, Laris B & Rolleri L (2006) *The impact of sex and HIV education programs in schools and communities on sexual behaviors among young adults*. New York: Research Triangle Park

Kirby D, Laris B & Rolleri L (2007) Sex and HIV education programs: Their impact on sexual behaviors of young people throughout the world. *Journal of Adolescent Health* 40(3): 206–217

KMOEST (Kenya Ministry of Education Science and Technology) (1997) Sessional Paper No. 4. Nairobi: Kenya Ministry of Education Science and Technology

KMOEST (2004) *Education Sector Policy on HIV and AIDS*. Nairobi: Kenya Ministry of Education Science and Technology

KMOEST (2005a) *Sessional paper No. 1 of 2005: A policy framework for education, training and research*. Nairobi: Kenya Ministry of Education Science and Technology

KMOEST (2005b) *Kenya education sector support program 2005–2010: Delivering quality education and training to all Kenyans*. Nairobi: Kenya Ministry of Education Science and Technology

KMOEST (2009) *Education facts and figures. Update 1 October 2009*. Nairobi: Kenya Ministry of Education Science and Technology

KNACC (Kenya National AIDS Control Council) (2005) *Kenyan National HIV/AIDS Strategic Plan 2005/6–2009/10*. Nairobi: Kenya National AIDS/STI Control Programme

KNACC (2009) *2007 Kenya AIDS indicator survey: Final report*. Nairobi: Kenya National AIDS/STI Control Programme

Lear D (1997) *Sex and sexuality; Risk and relationships and the age of AIDS*. London: Sage Publications

Leclerc-Madlala S (2002) On the virgin cleansing myth: Gendered bodies, AIDS and ethnomedicine. *African Journal of AIDS Research* 1(2): 87–95

Leclerc-Madlala S (2008) Age-disparate and intergenerational sex in southern Africa: The dynamics of hypervulnerability. AIDS 22: 17–22

MacKinnon C (1984) Not a moral. *Yale Law & Policy Review* 2(2): 321–345

Manda DK, Kimalu PK, Nafula NN & Kimani DN (2003) *Costs and benefits of eliminating child labour in Kenya*. KIPRA Working Paper No. 10, Institute for Policy Research and Analysis, Nairobi

Mathooko M (2009) Actualizing free primary education in Kenya for sustainable development. *The Journal of Pan African Studies* 2(8): 151–159

Messer LC, Shoe E, Canady M, Sheppard BK & Vincus A (2011) Reported adolescent sexual norms and the development of a social marketing campaign to correct youth misperceptions. *Journal of Children and Poverty* 17(1): 45–63

Millen DR (2000) *Rapid ethnography: Time-deepening strategies for HCI field research.* Paper presented at Designing Interactive Systems: Processes, Practices, Methods, And Techniques, August 2000, New York

Mirowski, J & Ross CE (2003) *Education, social status and health.* New York: Aldine de Gruyer

Mkumbo K & Ingham R (2010) What Tanzanian parents want (and do not want) covered in school-based sex and relationships education. *Sex Education* 10(1): 67–78

Mugimu CB & Nabadda R (2009) The role of pre-service and in-service teacher training (PITT) programmes in preparing teachers for HIV curriculum integration. *Prospects* 39(4): 383–397

Muraah WM & Kiarie WN (2001) *HIV and AIDS, facts that could change your life.* Nairobi: English Press

Mushi A, Armstrong-Schellenberg J, Mponda H & Lengeler C (2003) Targeted subsidy for malaria control with treated nets using a discount voucher system in southern Tanzania. *Health Policy and Planning* 18(2): 163–171

Mwale M (2009) Behavioural change vis-à-vis HIV & AIDS knowledge mismatch among adolescents. The case of some selected schools in Zomba, Malawi. *South African Journal of Psychology* 39(4): 460–467

Nieto S (1994) Lessons from students on creating a chance to dream. *Harvard Educational Review* 64(4): 392–426

Njue C, Nzioka C, Ahlberg B, Pertet AM & Voeten HACM (2009) 'If you don't abstain, you will die of AIDS': AIDS education in Kenyan schools. *AIDS Education and Prevention* 21(2): 169–179

Nyaga RK, Kimani DN, Mwabu G, Mwangi S & Kimenyi MS (2004) HIV/AIDS in Kenya: *A review of research and policy issues.* Discussion Paper No. 38, http://www.kippra.org/docs/DP38.pdf

Nykiel-Herbert B (2004) Mis-constructing knowledge: The case of learner-centred pedagogy in South Africa. *Prospects* 34(3): 249–265

Oakley A (1994) Women and children first and last. Parallels and differences between children's and women's studies. In B Mayall (Ed.) *Children's childhoods observed and experienced.* London: Falmer Press

Oliver D, Leeming F & Dwyer W (1998) Studying parental involvement in school-based sex education: Lessons learned. *Family Planning Perspectives* 30(3): 143–147

Oluga M, Kiragu S, Walli S & Mohamed M (2010) Deceptive cultural practices that sabotage HIV/AIDS education in Tanzania and Kenya. *Journal of Moral Education* 39(3): 365–380

Orner M (1996) Teaching for the moment: Intervention projects as situated pedagogy. *Theory into Practice* 35(2): 72–78

O-saki KM & Agu AO (2002) A study of classroom interaction in primary schools in the United Republic of Tanzania. *Prospects* 32(1): 102–116

O'Sullivan M (2004) The reconceptualisation of learner-centred approaches: a Namibian case study. *International Journal of Educational Development* 24(6): 585–602

Pattman R & Chege F (2003) *Finding our voices: Gendered and sexual identities and HIV/AIDS education.* Geneva: UNICEF

Perkins HW & Berkowitz A (1986) Perceiving the community norms of alcohol use among students: Some research implications for campus alcohol education programming. *International Journal of the Addictions* 21(9–10): 961–976

Plato & Grube GMA (2002) *Five dialogues: Euthyphro, Papology, Crito, Meno, Phaedo.* Indianapolis: Hackett Publishing

Pontefract C & Hardman F (2005) The discourses of classroom interactions in Kenyan primary schools. *Comparative Education* 42(1): 87–106

Prazak M (2000) Talking about sex: Construction of sexuality in rural Kenya. *Africa Today* 47(3/4): 83–97

Prophet RB & Rowell PM (1993) Coping and control: Science teaching strategies in Botswana. *Quality Studies in Education* 6: 197–209

Rivers K & Aggleton P (1999) *Adolescent sexuality, gender and the HIV epidemic.* New York: United Nations Development Programme

Rooth E (2005) *An investigation of the status and practice of life orientation in South African schools in two provinces.* Doctoral thesis, University of the Western Cape

Rudduck J (2005) *Pupil voice is here to stay!* London: Qualification and Curriculum Authority Futures

Rudduck J & Flutter J (2000) Pupil participation and pupil perspective: 'Carving a new order of experience'. *Cambridge Journal of Education* 30(1): 75–89

Rudduck J & McIntyre D (2007) *Improving learning through consulting pupils.* London: Routledge

Ryan K (1989) Sex, morals, and schools. *Theory into Practice* 28(3): 217–220

Scheerens J (2000) *Improving school effectiveness: Fundamentals of education planning No. 68.* Paris: UNESCO/ILEP

Scott D (2008) *Critical essays on major curriculum theorists.* London: Routledge

Shisana O, Rehle T, Simbayi LC, Zuma K, Jooste S et al. (2009) *South African national HIV prevalence, incidence, behaviour and communications survey 2008: A turning tide among teenagers?* Cape Town: HSRC Press

Shisana O, Simbayi L, Rehle T, Zungu N, Zuma K et al. (2010) *South African national HIV prevalence, incidence, behaviour and communication survey 2008: The health of our children.* Cape Town: HSRC Press

Shor I & Freire P (1987) A *pedagogy for liberation: Dialogues on transforming education.* London: Palgrave Macmillan

Simbayi L, Skinner D, Letlape L & Zuma K (Eds) (2005) *Workplace policies in public education: A review focusing on HIV/AIDS.* Cape Town: HSRC Press

Sinclair J & Coulthard M (1992) Towards an analysis of discourse. In M Coulthard (Ed.) *Advances in spoken discourse analysis.* London: Routledge

Siringi S (2002) East Africa to tackle high rates of child prostitution. *The Lancet* 359(9319): 1756

South Africa Department of Health (2007) *The Department of Health's national strategic plan for HIV and AIDS and sexually transmitted infections (STIs) 2007–2011.* Pretoria: DoH

South Africa Government Communication and Information Services (2009) *South Africa yearbook 2009/10.* Pretoria: GCIS

Statistics South Africa (2001) South African census 2001, http://www.statssa.gov.za/

Swartz S (2009) *The moral ecology of South Africa's township youth.* New York: Palgrave Macmillan

Swartz S (2011) 'Going deep' and 'giving back': Strategies for exceeding ethical expectations when researching among vulnerable youth. *Qualitative Research,* 11(1): 47–68

Swartz S & Bhana A (2009) *Teenage Tata: Voices of young fathers in South Africa.* Cape Town: HSRC Press

Tabulawa R (1997) Pedagogical classroom practice and the social context: The case of Botswana. *International Journal of Educational Development* 17(2): 189–204

Tanzania Commission for AIDS (2008) *Tanzania HIV/AIDS and malaria indicator survey 2007–2008.* Dar es Salaam: Commission for AIDS

Tanzania Ministry of Education and Culture (2000) *Secondary education master plan (SEMP) 2001–2005.* Dar es Salaam: Government Printer

Tanzania Ministry of Education and Culture (2004) *Strategic plan for HIV/AIDS 2003–2007.* Dar es Salaam: Tanzania Commission for AIDS

Tanzania Ministry of Educational and Vocational Training (2008) *Basic educational statistics in Tanzania.* Dar es Salaam: Ministry of Education and Vocational Training, http://moe.go.tz/statistics.html

Tanzania Prime Minister's Office (2001) *National policy on HIV/AIDS.* Government of Tanzania

Taylor N (2000) Schooling and everyday life. In J Muller (Ed.) *Reclaiming knowledge: Social theory curriculum and education policy.* London: Routledge Falmer

Tepper MS (2000) Sexuality and disability: The missing discourse of pleasure. *Sexuality and Disability* 18(4): 283–290

Terreblanche SJ (2002) *A history of inequality in South Africa, 1652–2002.* Pietermaritzburg: University of KwaZulu-Natal Press

TESDP (Tanzania Education Sector Development Program) (2009) *Education Sector Performance Report 2008/2009.* Tanzania: Education Sector Development Committee.

Thomson R & Scott L (1992) *An enquiry into sexuality education; report of a survey into local education and authority support and monitoring of school sexuality education.* London: National Children's Bureau.

Uganda AIDS Commission (2008) *National HIV & AIDS strategic plan 2007/8–2011/12. Moving towards universal access,* http://www.aidsuganda.org/IRC/documents/nsp.pdf

Umalusi (2004) *Investigation into the senior certificate examination: Summary report on the evaluation of the senior certificate examination August 2004.* Pretoria: Umalusi

UNAIDS/WHO (2009) *AIDS Epidemic update.* Geneva: Joint United Nations Programme on HIV/AIDS (UNAIDS)

UNAIDS/WHO (2010) *Global report: UNAIDS report on the global AIDS epidemic 2010.* Geneva: Joint United Nations Programme on HIV/AIDS (UNAIDS)

UNICEF (2010) *South Africa – Statistics,* http://www.unicef.org/infobycountry/southafrica_statistics.html#67

United Nations Integrated Regional Information Network (2006) *Free basic education the way forward.* Press clip from school fees workshop in Nairobi, 5 April. Copy in possession of author

UNSTATS (2005) United Nations Statistics Division, http://unstats.un.org

Van der Heijden I & Swartz S (2010) Bereavement, silence and culture within a peer-led HIV/AIDS-prevention strategy for vulnerable children in South Africa. *African Journal of AIDS Research* 9(1): 41–50

Vavrus F (2009) The cultural politics of constructivist pedagogies: Teacher education reform in the United Republic of Tanzania. *International Journal of Educational Development* 29(3): 303–311

Verspoor AD (Ed.) (2003) *The challenge of learning – improving basic education in sub-Saharan Africa.* Paris: Association for the Development of Education in Africa (ADEA)

Vygotsky LS (1978) *Mind and society: The development of higher mental processes.* Cambridge, MA: Harvard University Press

Wambuii HK (2006) *The politics of HIV/AIDS and implications for democracy in Kenya.* New York: The Edwin Mellen Press

Wang C & Burris MA (1994) Empowerment through photovoice: Portraits of participation. *Health Education Quarterly* 21(2): 171–186

Wang C & Burris MA (1997) Photovoice: Concept, methodology, and use for participatory needs assessment. *Health Education & Behavior* 24(3): 367–387

Wedgwood R (2005) Post-basic education and poverty in Tanzania. Post-Basic Education and Training Working Paper Series No. 1, Centre of African Studies, University of Edinburgh

White A (2003) The application of Sinclair and Coulthard's IRF structure to a classroom lesson: Analysis and discussion, http://www.cels.bham.ac.uk/resources/essays/AWhite4.pdf.

Wilton T (1997) *Engendering AIDS: Deconstructing sex, text and epidemic.* London: Sage Publications

World Bank (2002) *Education and HIV/AIDS: A window of hope.* Washington, DC: World Bank

World Bank (2003) Education: The social vaccine to HIV/AIDS, http//go.worldbank.org/VSUKCHBJO

World Bank (2006) *Tanzania country report context.* Washington, DC: World Bank

Yu W (2009) An analysis of college English classroom discourse. *Asian Social Science* 7(5), www.ccsenet.org/journal.html

Zisser A & Francis D (2006) Youth have a new attitude on AIDS, but are they talking about it? *African Journal of AIDS Research* 5(2): 189–196

Appendix 1: Research instruments

Rapid ethnography

Observation sheets (5–7 days, helpful to include a weekend)

Aim: To write a 5–10-page background piece on 'What's going on in this school?'
Basic demographic information.

School
1. Poverty levels: Do children come to school hungry? Do they travel long distances to get to school?
2. School climate: Is the school organised or not?
3. Attendance: Are children disciplined or not? Do they come to school regularly for the whole day or play truant? What is the atmosphere in the classroom like? Is there controlled discussion and general happiness or do teachers struggle to maintain control?
4. Playground: Is there fear or happiness at school?
5. Are there any irregular relationships between teachers and students in this school?
6. What's the school's academic performance like?

Home
7. What kinds of homes do children live in – flats, huts, houses? What do we learn about poverty levels from this?
8. Are both parents present in the household? Who do children come home to after school?

Community
9. What are the prevailing views in the community (Christian, Muslim, traditional, modern)?
10. Are people working, employed?
11. Is the community a 'village' i.e. other parents look out for children, or do neighbours know each other?
12. Is there *ubuntu*, *ujamaa*, collectivism, neighbourliness?
13. Is there crime, lots of young people in jail, in gangs?

Streets (youth culture)
14. What are the recreational practices of the children?
15. What are the streets like during the day, at night?

Children

Individual interview 1: Sources of sexual knowledges (15–20 minutes)

Photovoice project 1:

(For the young people chosen). Take a maximum of 10 photographs of the places and/or people where you get your information about sex, AIDS and romantic relationships, e.g. the home, the local meeting place (This task is given to the young people during the week of rapid ethnography and they have two weeks to complete it.)

1. What is this picture?
2. Tell me how you get the information from this source (e.g. television).
3. What does this source teach you?
   Probes: Sex, AIDS, relationships
4. Tell me some of the differences between each of these sources.
   Is it different for sex/relationships/AIDS?
5. Which source is most important to you? Why?
   Rank them 1–10
6. Which is most helpful to you?
   Can you give me an example of how this source has helped you?
7. Can you give me an example of some occasion where you needed information and didn't have it about sex/AIDS/relationships?
8. What picture did you want to take but weren't able to?

Individual interview 2: School AIDS education and gender, religion and culture (15–20 minutes)

1. Tell me about the AIDS education you receive at school?
   Probes: What do they teach you, how do they teach it?
2. What do you think about what they teach you?
   Probes: Is it boring, is it exciting, is it embarrassing, are they in touch with the reality of being young in Kenya/South Africa/Tanzania?
3. Can you give me an example of something you learnt at school that you implemented in your life?
4. Can you give me an example where something you learnt at school clashed with what someone else told you about sex, AIDS or relationships?
5. How does what you believe (religion) affect your view of AIDS education?
6. How do your traditional beliefs (culture) affect your view of AIDS education?
7. How does being a young man/young woman affect your response to AIDS education?
8. What are the characteristics of AIDS education that you'd like to see in school?

Focus group discussion: What is right/wrong with school AIDS education? (30 mins)

Project 2:

Create two short documentaries (using the video on the cameras) of no longer than two minutes each that show how AIDS education is:
- currently taught to you at school (current practice);
- and how you'd like it to be taught (desired practice).

Invite research participants to meet, show the documentaries and discuss them in a focus group that asks the following:
1. How realistic is this documentary (current practice)?
2. What features does this documentary highlight?
3. Is there anything with which you disagree?
4. What has been left out?
5. How realistic is this documentary (desired practice)?
6. What features does this documentary highlight?
7. Is there anything with which you disagree?
8. What has been left out?

Teachers

Individual interview (15 mins)
1. Tell me a story or describe an incident when you believed you were doing effective AIDS education?
2. Tell me about a time when you felt prevented from teaching about AIDS in a way you believed would be effective?

If an AIDS education lesson was observed then ask:
3. What were the key moments in this AIDS lesson? How did you know you were being effective?

Focus group discussion (30–45 mins)
1. What AIDS education occurs in your school?
2. What training for AIDS education have you received?
3. How do you feel about teaching AIDS education at school?
4. What are the struggles and challenges you face in teaching AIDS education?
   Dilemmas and problems:
5. How do you think various factors affect how AIDS education is done in schools?
   a. Culture
   b. Religion
   c. Gender
   d. Being an adult
   e. Being a teacher
6. Can you give me any examples of ways in which you've used students' 'everyday knowledge' in your teaching practice?

Show AIDS education documentaries – desired version.
7. What do you think of students' desired vision for school AIDS education?
   a. What is realistic, not realistic?
   b. What small steps could you take to realise this vision?

Community stakeholders

Individual interview (15 minutes)

Religious leader, parent, grandparent, school head, traditional healer, medical person, NGO worker
1. How do you think our culture affects what AIDS education is done in schools?
2. How do you think our religion affects what AIDS education is done in schools?
3. What do you think the role of the school should be in educating young people about AIDS?
4. What advice do you have for me about (teaching) AIDS education in schools?

Community dialogue

Focus group discussion (2 hours)

Groups of teachers, pupils, school principals, religious leaders, parents, traditional leaders/healers, and other stakeholders per school

Welcome and ground rules (15 minutes)

Everyone's opinion is important. There are no teachers or pupils today, just participants. Thank every-one for participating. Give cameras to schools as a token of appreciation.

Young people's sexual knowledges (45 minutes)

Show extracts from the photovoice activity from all three countries.
1. What do you think of the data you have heard and seen? Are you surprised, not surprised, shocked, angered, pleased?
2. Will it make you do anything differently?
3. Do you think we should use young people's knowledge as part of HIV/AIDS and sex education? If so, how?

If they said yes then we asked:
4. How do you think it can be used?
5. What are the challenges of using young people's sexual knowledges in school? (We were looking to explore the social, educational and personal challenges.)

Sex education (45 minutes)

Watch the desired videos from all three countries. Then take 10 minutes to answer the questions below in writing.
6. What do you notice as the main things that students want?
7. What do you think of the students' views?
8. How is teaching about sex and AIDS different from other teaching for teachers?
9. How do you think we should decide what is in sex- and HIV/AIDS-education classes and how should it be taught?
10. Should we create an atmosphere or climate in which teachers and students can talk honestly to each other? If so, how?

11. What sort of support do schools need to work differently?
12. Are there cultural and religious issues about dealing with sex and HIV/AIDS? How should schools deal with them?

Group dialogue (15 minutes)

Group provides feedback on their experiences of participating in the dialogues.

FLANDERS INTERACTION ANALYSIS SYSTEM OBSERVATION SHEET

Observation of setting

Date	Time	Class	Lesson / activity		Length of observation

		Every 2–5 minutes																			
Teacher talk	Direct	Accepts feelings Praises or encourages Accepts/uses students' ideas Asks questions																			
	Indirect	Lectures Gives direction Criticises or justifies authority																			
Student talk		Response																			
		Initiation																			
Silence, confusion or uncodeable																					

Appendix 2: Toolkit for change

This appendix provides a text version of the electronic toolkit available to practitioners at http://www. educ.cam.ac.uk/centres/cce/initiatives/projects/askaids/publications.html.The toolkit has three aims:

1. To help practitioners set up a consultation process regarding sex and AIDS education with children, teachers and stakeholders
2. To develop a hybrid sex education curriculum for children
3. To support a process of continuous improvement with regard to sex and AIDS education in the classroom

Acknowledgements

We would like to thank the individuals and organisations that enabled this research to take place. The researchers came from three institutions and we thank them: The Centre for Commonwealth Education, Faculty of Education, University of Cambridge, Cambridge, UK, which funded the research; the Human Sciences Research Council, Cape Town, South Africa; and the Aga Khan University Institute for Educational Development (East Africa), Dar es Salaam, Tanzania. We would also like to thank Duncan Scott and Busi Magazi at the HSRC, who gave of their time and effort in collecting and managing the data and writing, as did Mary Cobbett at the Commonwealth Centre for Education, who helped in the final stages.

We thank the ministries and departments of education in Kenya, South Africa and Tanzania for giving permission for this research. We owe the greatest thanks to the teachers, students and stakeholders in the schools we worked in. Research makes great demands on colleagues in schools and we are grateful for their time and cooperation.

How to use this toolkit

The idea of this toolkit is to help you develop your HIV/AIDS education by consulting your pupils about what they know about HIV/AIDS and how they want HIV/AIDS education to be taught. You can use it:

1. On your own
2. With a colleague
3. With a group of interested teachers

We have provided ideas not only to help you consult pupils and community members, but also ideas to help your learning and reflection on your own practice. So there are quizzes, readings and activities. We suggest you keep a journal of what you are doing in order to monitor your own progress. The sections included in the toolkit are:

1. A background of the problem of HIV/AIDS in sub-Saharan Africa
2. Key findings from our research
3. Why teachers and practitioners should consult pupils
4. Tools and activities for consultation with young people and stakeholders
5. How we used these activities in our research
6. A final reflection

Background to HIV/AIDS in sub-Saharan Africa

Sub-Saharan Africa remains the region of the world most severely impacted upon by HIV/AIDS. In 2008, sub-Saharan Africa reported 67 per cent of HIV/AIDS infections worldwide, 68 per cent of new HIV/AIDS infections among adults (with 40 per cent of all new infections being among children aged 15 and over), and 91 per cent of new HIV/AIDS infections among children.

Fourteen million children have been orphaned in sub-Saharan Africa, and 72 per cent of the world's HIV/AIDS-related deaths are located here. The situation is worse for girls and young women. In Kenya, young women between 15 and 19 years are three times more likely to be infected than males, and 20- to 24-year-old women are 5.5 times more likely to be living with HIV/AIDS than men in their age group. Among people aged 15 to 24 living in Tanzania, females are four times more likely than males to be living with HIV/AIDS. Women are more vulnerable because of their limitation to negotiate when, how and where to have sex. Biologically, their sexual reproductive system makes infection more likely than in men. Heterosexual intercourse remains the primary mode of HIV/AIDS transmission in sub-Saharan Africa, as well as the primary transmission of the disease to newborns and breastfed babies. HIV/AIDS is also transmitted through needle sharing and among men who have unprotected sex with men.

HIV/AIDS and education

Education has proven to be vital in the fight against HIV/AIDS, as educated young people have lower rates of infection. Better education among girls has been particularly important in this regard, since rates of infection among teenage girls are five times higher than boys. Thus, HIV-prevention education has become known as the 'social vaccine'. Uganda is a good example of how HIV/AIDS-related education in formal schooling, as well as community education programmes, reduced prevalence rates from 18 per cent in 1992 to 6 per cent in 2002. Governments have introduced HIV-related educational programmes that include life skills, reproductive health programmes and other health interventions in schools. HIV/AIDS has had a big impact on pupils and teachers. Pupils have lost their parents to the disease, and schools are facing the challenge of dealing with orphans and consequent high dropout rates among orphans who have lost one or both parents to the disease. Teachers have also been infected and are dying faster than they can be replaced.

Toolkit activity: Test your knowledge

Study the table below dealing with HIV/AIDS statistics in sub-Saharan Africa and fill in the missing words in the next section.

	Adults and children living with HIV	Adults and children newly infected with HIV	Percentage adult prevalence (15 to 49 years)	AIDS-related deaths among adults and children
2009	22.5 million (20.9–24.2 million)	1.8 million (1.6–2.0 million)	5.0 (4.7–5.2)	1.3 million (1.1–1.5 million)
2001	20.3 million (18.9–21.7 million)	2.2 million (1.9–2.4 million)	5.9 (5.6–6.1)	1.4 million (1.2–1.6 million)

See our website for the full UNAIDS/WHO (2010) report on the global AIDS epidemic, http://www.educ.cam.ac.uk/centres/cce/initiatives/projects/askaids/publications.html

Based on information from the previous page and the table above, read the paragraph below and fill in the missing words.

An estimated _____ million adults and children were living with HIV in sub-Saharan Africa at the end of 2009. This was a decrease of _____ million people from 2001. In 2009, _____ of adults aged 15 to 49 years were HIV-positive and _____ million people died of AIDS-related illnesses. Overall, the rate of new infections has gone down from _____ million in 2001 to _____ million in 2009.

Based on information from the previous page and the table above, reflect on the questions below:

1. Why do you think the number of people infected with HIV/AIDS increased from 20.3 million in 2001 to 22.5 million in 2009?
2. Why do you think the number of new infections fell from 2.2 million in 2001 to 1.8 million in 2009?
3. Why do you think that more females than males are infected with HIV/AIDS in sub-Saharan Africa?
4. What problems do you think the 14 million orphaned children in sub-Saharan Africa face?

Toolkit reflection: Knowing the facts

In your journal, please comment on the following:

1. Do you know the statistics concerning HIV/AIDS in your immediate community? Where could you find this information?
2. Walk around your community. Do you see any HIV/AIDS information on public display? If yes, do you think it is clear and adequate?
3. How often do you and your family, friends and colleagues at work discuss HIV/AIDS? Should you be the one who starts and/or supports these conversations? Do you feel that you have the facts right?
4. What are the myths about HIV/AIDS in your community?

Key findings from our research

The content of this toolkit was informed by a research study funded by the Commonwealth Education Trust. It took place in Kenya, South Africa and Tanzania, and involved 130 pupils and 48 teachers. Key findings from this study are presented below in three themes: young people's sexual knowledges, sexual education in schools and dialogue about the data.

On young people's sexual knowledges

- Young people have wide-ranging and fairly sophisticated knowledge of adults' sexual practices and sexual worlds, e.g. prostitution, the influence of drugs and alcohol, and rape.
- They observe sexual acts regularly and are well aware of the particular practices in their environs.
- The young people were primary-aged pupils in this study, so we can assume that this occurs at a fairly young age.
- They are well aware of the consequences of unprotected sex and HIV/AIDS and are keen to avoid them.
- They want a lot more information and dialogue with adults on sexual matters and HIV/AIDS in particular.
- They are aware that they cannot share this knowledge with adults and that adults are ambivalent and avoid talking to young people honestly and openly about sexual matters and HIV/AIDS.
- There is a difference between what girls and boys experience. While there are gender differences, there are also common cross-gender concerns.

On sex education in schools

- Young people want a more interactive and active pedagogy that allows them to engage with their own knowledge and talk about their lack of knowledge.
- They are concerned that the information they get is unrealistic and does not reflect the world in which they live.
- Teachers want to help but not many are confident or feel well resourced. Some are more frightened of engaging in discussions about HIV/AIDS than others – especially a fear of parents and community leaders.
- The school or the practices in school are influenced by the wider community and the dominant attitudes (e.g. religion, cultural practices). The school is a mirror of the community in which it is located.
- There are very different conceptions about the values and approaches that might be effective and which of these should be adopted.

Dialogue about the data

In our research we proposed that a way to shift attitudes and engage with the sexual knowledge of young people might be to share the findings of the data on young people's sexual knowledge and their preferred form of sex education. This we did and we found that:

- Adults (teachers, parents and community leaders) were surprised at and interested in the extent and nature of the young people's knowledge.
- Adults were willing to engage with the idea of non-naïve young people and this fact offered a different possibility in terms of sex and HIV/AIDS education.
- Adults seemed open to the potential for dialogue about HIV/AIDS education for their young people.

Why teachers and practitioners should consult pupils

There are various reasons why we should consult pupils when it comes to HIV/AIDS and sex education. First, we know HIV/AIDS education works, and that it requires a participatory teaching and learning method to develop understanding among teachers, parents and their children. That is why we have created this toolkit for teachers' use. For example, in Zimbabwe, a recent study showed that HIV prevalence rates were much lower among 15- to 19-year-olds who were attending school. This tells us that formal education may have a protective role. Similar results were found in 15- to 24-year-olds in southern Africa, especially among girls who typically have five times the infection rate as similar-aged boys. We believe formal education can work as a social vaccine. Education is very powerful in helping to reduce rates of HIV/AIDS, but unfortunately many HIV/AIDS-education programmes have been biological (fact-based) and have lacked connections to young people's social and lived experiences. When young people cannot relate school-based HIV/AIDS education to their lives and experiences, the impact is limited.

Second, young people have often asked for recognition, saying there is a big gap between the education they need and what is being provided by their parents and educators. They want the opportunity, within open dialogue, to learn about the emotional implications of relationships as well as the biology of sex and sexual health promotion. They want a chance to talk about the problem and the disease. Research has found that pupils have much to say about their teaching and learning. When their perspectives are taken seriously they feel more positive about themselves as learners, can understand and manage their own progress better, and feel more included in the school's aims. They believe that what they say makes a difference. The teachers involved in consulting with pupils also find it beneficial; it helps them understand how to support pupil engagement and build more open, collaborative and communicative relationships with their pupils. To achieve this, it would be helpful if teachers consulted their pupils on their knowledges and needs.

Research suggests (see additional readings below) that it is productive for teachers to consult with pupils and talk with them about things that really matter. This may involve:

- conversations about teaching and learning;
- seeking advice from pupils about new initiatives;
- inviting comments on ways of solving problems that are affecting the teacher's right to teach and the pupil's right to learn; and
- inviting evaluative comments on recent developments in school or classroom policy and practice.

Consultation on the part of the teachers must be genuine and provide the opportunity to hear from silent or silenced pupils. This would help in understanding why some disengage and what would help them get back on track. (See the guidelines for consultation) below. Honest consultation is not easy because it challenges traditional power relationships. Some teachers feel that pupils are too young and inexperienced to voice anything worthwhile. Teachers may also feel that there is little time to consult pupils, or they may be uncertain about the process of consultation. However, researchers note that perhaps the most important principle for teachers to follow is to help pupils to feel:

- they really have a voice;
- they are listened to; and
- they matter.

Teachers are potentially one of the most important tools in HIV/AIDS education. Research tells us teachers can become these important tools when they engage in consultative learning and teaching. Not only does this approach enhance sustainability of positive teacher-pupil relationships, but it also builds capacity among the teachers to support pupil learning.

Preparing to consult pupils

Before you use this toolkit or commence any activities with your pupils, you need to think carefully about your school setting and the pupils in your care. Consider these questions and talk with your colleagues and your head teacher or school principal to gain an understanding of where you work and what goes on there. The exercise that follows will help you better understand your pupils' contexts so that you will be able to more knowledgably teach and help your pupils.

Toolkit activity: Reflecting on pupils' lives and contexts

1. Poverty levels: Do children come to school hungry? Do they travel far to get to school?
2. Attendance: Do children come to school regularly, for the whole day or part?
3. What is the atmosphere in the classroom like?
4. What methods of teaching and learning are used?
5. What is play or break time like?
6. What is the relationship between pupils and teachers like?
7. How does the situation above affect children's learning?
8. What are the prevailing views on HIV/AIDS and sexuality in the community?
9. How do people in the community spend their time?
10. Is there *ubuntu*, *ujamaa*, collectivism, neighbourliness?
11. Is there sex education in the community?

12. What are the recreational practices of the children?
13. What are the streets like during the day, at night?
14. How would you describe young people's lives in your community?

Guidelines for consultation

Once you have understood pupils' contexts, you can now explore how to make use of the activities in this toolkit for effective participatory teaching in your HIV/AIDS-education lessons. Below are a few basic guidelines for consultation that we suggest you and your pupils follow. Before sharing these rules with your pupils, spend some time letting pupils suggest some rules. Let them generate as many as they can. Write them down on the chalkboard or on a flip chart. When they have exhausted their ideas, share with them guidelines from the list below. There is no need to repeat those already mentioned by the pupils.

1. Explain to your pupils that they will all be involved in the consultation.
2. Explain to them that 'many heads' are better than one. In other words – one finger alone cannot kill a louse any more than one stone can hold a cooking pot. That's the basic idea behind consultation – all of us are smarter than one of us alone.
3. Remind them that every idea should be respected – no laughing at other's ideas and be respectful when presenting your idea so that you don't offend others.
4. Remind your pupils that they must be courteous if they want to become respected members in the consultation.
5. Remember, not everyone immediately feels comfortable working with others. Trust comes from experience – it is earned not expected.
6. Remind pupils that what is said in the class stays in the class. Then, if the class agrees, their statements could be shared in the larger community – no individual names get used!
7. All contributions to the class discussion should be consultative.
8. Every member of the class must make an active contribution to the discussion. No one should get a 'free ride'.
9. Whenever possible, class members should find evidence to add to the discussion. Facts rather than rumours strengthen the contributions.
10. Make sure the class understands how much time there is available for the activity.
11. Make sure the class knows what you hope the outcome will be and why their involvement in the consultative process is important.

For more guidance on how to work ethically with your pupils, please see our website, www.educ.cam.ac.uk/centres/cce/askaids

Tools and activities for consultation with young people

The first step is to ensure that you are following the 'Guidelines for consultation' outlined above. The next step is to decide what you want to consult on and how. The following pages provide a basket of tools that can be used for consultation. See below for more information on each of our tools. After the tools have been presented, the next section 'How we used these activities in our research' describes how we used some of the tools. Suggestions are then given for how some of the tools can be used for different purposes under the following headings:

Tool 1: Consulting pupils about their sources of sexual knowledge
Tool 2: Consulting pupils about the HIV/AIDS and sex education they want
Tool 3: Working with community members
Tool 4: Working with fellow teachers

Focus groups

Focus groups are a way of getting a group of young people to share their ideas together and to help them build on each other's ideas. Please refer to the suggestions offered in 'Guidelines for consultation' for more information.

Materials needed
- Paper with questions to guide each group's discussion
- Pencil and paper to record significant discussion points

Instructions
- It might be better to have single-sex groups, i.e. all girls together or all boys together.
- Decide what key questions you want to ask beforehand.
- Ask the questions and let the group talk among themselves.
- You can use general statements such as 'We know all we need to know about HIV/AIDS – how best can we do this?' or 'We would like a different sort of HIV/AIDS education in our school – what should change?'.
- Alternatively, you could make up your own questions. Questions should be open-ended to allow for discussion.
- Decide how you will record the answers. Will you tape or digitally record them or take notes?
- If you are taking notes, ask the group if your notes are correct by checking the main points with them at the end.

We have suggested some more questions which you can use in this activity in the section 'Tool 1: Consulting pupils on the sources of their sexual knowledge'.

Suggestion box

Pupils may be embarrassed to ask some personal or sensitive questions, or may fear repercussions if they give critical feedback. A suggestion box is a safe way for them to drop in any questions or comments, or to share their concerns. It is anonymous and confidential and thus may encourage pupils to ask about anything at any convenient time.

Materials needed
- A suggestion box. This could use local resources or recycled material like a sealed wooden box, old suitcase, sealed cardboard box, etc. – with a slot where the pupils drop their comments
- Pencil and paper

Instructions
- Get the suggestion box and label it.
- Put the suggestion box in a prominent place in the classroom. You can negotiate with the pupils where it is best to place it.
- Explain that they are welcome to give any feedback or ask questions about HIV/AIDS-related issues.
- Instruct them not to write their names, but that they are welcome to indicate their age and sex.
- Allow them to use the language that they are most comfortable with.
- Agree on when they would like their questions to be answered and by whom (depending on whether there's another appropriate person available).

We have suggested some questions which you can use in this activity in the section 'Tool 2: Consulting pupils about the HIV/AIDS and sex education they want'.

Group survey

A survey can be used to ascertain what pupils know or to rate the quality of an HIV/AIDS lesson. A survey can be done at the beginning, middle and end of the term to monitor change in knowledges and lesson quality.

Materials needed
- A questionnaire, either closed or open ended
- Pens and pencils

Instructions
- Distribute the questionnaires to pupils and give them time to answer the questions.
- You can either tally the responses yourself or allow the pupils to exchange questionnaires among them so as to tally themselves – for a knowledge-based survey. You will have to read out the answers to them. For a quality evaluation you might allow pupils to discuss results in groups and come up with a consensus view, then report back to the class.

We have suggested some questions which you can use in this activity in the section 'Tool 1: Consulting pupils about their sources of sexual knowledge'.

Spot check

A spot check activity can give the teacher instant feedback on the efficacy of his/her approach. It helps you evaluate pupils' motivation, concentration, understanding and engagement with the lesson.

Materials needed
- Paper
- Pens and pencils

Instructions
- List the attributes you want to spot-check, e.g. concentration level, interest level, relevant to me, not relevant to me, wanting to ask a question or not.
- Do the spot check.
- Rate the observation from 1–4, with 4 being the best rating.
- Feedback to the pupils and discuss the situation, e.g. if the pupils are tired and sleepy, is it because they are hungry? If they are silent, is it because the lesson is too abstract?

Drawing

Drawing activities often help pupils to express themselves if they lack the vocabulary or are shy or afraid to talk about issues that are sensitive or culturally taboo.

Materials needed

- Pencils
- Paintbrushes
- Paint – several colours
- Newsprint, flip chart or manila paper
- Tape
- Containers (recycled tins, etc.) for the paint and water

Instructions

- Pupils can draw posters of what they want to know or of what they know about HIV/AIDS and sex.
- Each group should create a poster on the flip chart paper provided for this activity.

Please refer to the suggestions offered in 'Guidelines for consultation' for more information. We have suggested some questions which you can use in this activity in the section 'Tool 1: Consulting pupils about their sources of sexual knowledge'.

Role play

Role plays are effective in finding out what young people know and want. You could ask them to role play a typical dilemma about HIV/AIDS and sex, or role play what sort of HIV/AIDS education they want and have now. Please refer to the suggestions offered in 'Guidelines for consultation' for more information.

Materials needed

None

Instructions

- Organise the pupils into groups.
- Discuss the theme of the play with the pupils.
- Brainstorm the various roles they might play, and how these roles illustrate the theme of the play.
- Tell the pupils how long they have to create the play, organise themselves and be ready to perform.
- Leave the pupils to come up with the storyline and share out the roles.
- When they are ready (and within the allocated time) the pupils should present the role play to the rest of the class.
- After watching the role play, the class can ask the group questions. This could be an entry point to a class discussion.
- You, the teacher, should debrief the role-play activity using the following questions:

1. How realistic was this role play?
2. What features does this role play highlight?
3. Is there anything with which you disagree?
4. What has been left out?

See the videos (on our website) in 'How we used these activities in our research', especially the section entitled 'Pupils' suggestions of the HIV/AIDS education they want to receive'. They are examples of role plays done by the pupils in our research study.

Pupil-to-pupil interviews

In this activity pupils become their own researchers. This activity should be done after extensive group work. For this activity to be successful, a high level of trust must be established among the pupils. Please refer to the suggestions offered in 'Guidelines for consultation' for more information.

Materials needed
- Paper with questions to guide each group's discussion
- Pencil and paper to record significant discussion points

Instructions
- Organise pupils into pairs
- Assign one to be the interviewer and the other to be the interviewee
- Eventually the pupils should swap roles so that each asks the same questions
- Record the responses
- Present the findings to the class

We have suggested some questions which you can use in this activity in the section 'Tool 2: Consulting pupils about the HIV/AIDS and sex education they want'.

Voting cards

Teachers can also get pupils to vote and rate the quality of the class. Give the pupils paper or cards and ask them to rate the quality of the lesson, e.g. Did they enjoy it? Did they find it relevant? They can score from 1–4, with 4 being the highest vote. The results can be used as an entry point to discuss how to improve the lesson further.

Materials needed
- Squares of paper or cards, one per evaluation statement
- Pen and pencils

Instructions
- Distribute papers/cards to pupils.
- Ask them to rate the lesson from 1–4, with 4 being the best rating.
- Ask them to hold up their cards one at a time and you will see the rating.
- Alternatively, they can drop their cards in a 'ballot box' or hand them over to one pupil who will tally the votes for you and feed back the results to the class.

Working with student representatives and stakeholders

Set up a group consisting of pupils and stakeholders to dialogue about HIV/AIDS and sex education, and other related issues in the school and community. This will sensitise the relevant adults on what the children know about HIV/AIDS and also how they want HIV/AIDS and sex education to be improved. Dialogue within this group would then focus on how to develop the current HIV/AIDS education offered with the aim to make it more relevant to the pupils – with due consideration for their street, religious and indigenous cultures. We have suggested some questions which you can use in this activity in the sections 'Tool 3: Working with community members' and 'Tool 4: Working with fellow teachers'.

Photography

This activity can be done by the teacher and pupils. If you have a camera, you can take photos of the pupils doing the activities mentioned above. (If this is for research purposes you will need the permission of both the child and his/her guardian.) You could also take a photograph of any examples of interactive learning in the classroom, and of anything new and different happening in your HIV/AIDS-education lesson. The pupils, too, can have access to the camera and can be tasked to take pictures on themes related to HIV/AIDS, e.g. their sources of sexual knowledges, challenges in their community. The photos can be discussed in the classroom with the pupils. With pupils' permission, the photos may be discussed with other relevant stakeholders.

Materials needed
- Camera(s)
- Batteries
- Memory cards

Instructions
- For teachers – take photos of new practices in your HIV/AIDS lessons.
- For pupils – take photos of a theme discussed with the teacher.
- The teacher's and pupils' photos will be entry points to discussions.

We have suggested some questions which you can use in this activity in the section 'Tool 1: Consulting pupils on the sources of their sexual knowledge'.

How we used these activities in our research

We used many of these activities in our research study. Below we describe how we used some of these activities to consult pupils about the sources and content of their sexual knowledges.

Sources of sexual knowledges

Children get their sexual knowledges from various sources in both the formal and informal settings of their lives. The video you are going to see presents some insights to these sources. The school, as a formal source of knowledge, has wall paintings encouraging pupils to avoid drug abuse and abstain from sex, including intergenerational sex. They also get similar information from, among others, teachers, peers, books and speakers. However, the pupils are exposed to these very things in their home environments. They see sex, prostitution and drug abuse. For example, in our research, Juma, a 12-year-old boy from School A in Tanzania, explained how smoking marijuana had made youth in his village 'get euphoric effects which lead them into doing sex'. Binti (12 years old) and Dalila (12 years old), two girls from School C in Kenya, had seen sexual intercourse live in the public spaces of their neighbourhood as a result of drug intoxication:

Binti: When they inhale these substances…they don't wait to get a room. They get any man and start having sex in public…there and then, at the point of contact.
Researcher: Have you seen this?
Binti: I see them…outside our house…in the football field. Especially on Saturday and Sunday the field is packed. The prostitutes, the drunkards…
Researcher: It means the children have already seen sex!
Binti: Children know what sex is because they see it.

Dalila: It is the norm to make love in the open…even as cars pass by. They do it there and then. They do not go to hidden places, they do not fear…they have drunk and used drugs, they will not care who sees them.

Naledi, a 13-year-old girl from School A, South Africa, said that children already knew about sex: 'We see it on TV; and some of us are already doing it.' Everyday habits, such as shaving and washing, also pose a risk, as pupils in poor communities may share razor blades, toothbrushes and wash sponges. Young people's photographs abound with images of these artefacts.

As you watch the video, think about the following questions:
1. What information is represented in these photos? For example, correct or incorrect knowledge, formal or informal knowledge?
2. Which forms of information might be more powerful to boys or to girls?
3. How can they (in-school and out-of-school knowledges) work together?

Toolkit reflection: Sources of sexual knowledge

Take some time to reflect on what you have just learned. With a colleague discuss the following questions:
1. What are the different sources of sexual knowledges in your community?
2. Which sources seem more powerful?

In your journal describe what you think of the children's images of their sexual worlds. What are the challenges they face in sorting out the different and often competing forms of knowledge they encounter?

See our website to see examples of the photographs that children took showing their sources of sexual knowledge, as well as some of the other tools we used to obtain this information, http://www.educ.cam.ac.uk/centres/cce/initiatives/projects/askaids/publications.html

Pupils' perceptions of the HIV/AIDS-related education they receive

In many schools, HIV/AIDS education is offered through formal instructional programmes that provide young people with information on human development, emotions and relationships, self-esteem, sexual health, sexual behaviour and sexual violence. Pupils are very clear about the kind of information they want and need. Please watch the video available on our website and listen closely to what the children are saying. Consider what pupils think about the HIV/AIDS-related education they receive. Also see our website for videos about the HIV/AIDS education that pupils want.

Pupils' suggestions on the HIV/AIDS-related education they want to receive

In contrast to the often practised didactic teaching method, as shown in pupils' videos regarding the current sex education they receive, young people have expressed the wish to have a comprehensive approach to HIV/AIDS education. They want their parents and teachers to talk to them about sexual matters and HIV and AIDS without feeling embarrassed. This approach recognises young people as worthy decision-makers, especially if given the opportunity to access good information. Though abstinence is desirable, the comprehensive approach to HIV/AIDS-related education recognises young people's right to information and acknowledges them as sexual beings. As such, it is imperative to provide open knowledge and skills about issues of sexuality. HIV/AIDS-related education does not increase sexual activity. Pupils want the pedagogy for HIV/AIDS-related education to be more active and interactive through role plays and games, videos, opportunities to explore dilemmas, practising communication, discussions that are open and come from multiple perspectives (including cultural). They also want talks from visitors, such as those living with HIV or AIDS, and young parents. Further suggestions included having a comments-and-suggestion box prominently placed in the classroom to allow pupils, who might otherwise feel embarrassed, to ask questions and have a chance to say what they want to learn about. They also want to know more about puberty and body changes, sex and relationships, peer-pressure problems, same-sex relationships, contraception, STIs, HIV, pros and cons about sex, when is the right time to have sex and where to get advice. Just from these views offered by the pupils in our study, it is possible to see that these children, if given the opportunity, have worthwhile contributions to make with regard to what HIV/AIDS and sex education should entail.

See our website to watch the video about how role playing can make teaching more active and children more engaged in their learning.

Toolkit reflection: Teaching practice

In your journal, reflect on your own teaching practice by answering the following questions:
1. To what degree does your teaching practice actively involve students?
2. Are your lessons participatory?
3. What are the children doing with the information you give them?
4. How are the children demonstrating to you that they have learned the information you are teaching?
5. What do you find hard to discuss in class?
6. How might you use indirect methods, e.g. case studies or fictional stories to help stimulate discussions where participants do not feel exposed?

Find a colleague who is interested in working with you to improve your teaching practice and your classroom environment.
1. Ask your colleague to watch you teach.
2. Use the journal prompts above as a way of analysing your teaching practice.
3. Trade places with your colleague and watch him or her teach.
4. Discuss what you have seen and identify areas for improvement.

See our website for the tools that were used to consult pupils about the HIV/AIDS and sex education they want.

Tool 1: Consulting pupils about their sources of sexual knowledge

Q. How can you (the teacher) find out from the children their sources of sexual knowledges?

Suggested activities and guiding questions – refer to the previous topic ' Tools and activities for consultation with young people' for further guidance. Choose from them and from some of the questions below.

Focus group discussions

1. Is there anything in your *neighbourhood* that has given you information on or reminded you of HIV/AIDS, drugs and sex? If yes, please explain.
    *   If a person or people, who are they and what did they do or say?
    *   If an object, picture or book, what is it and what was its message?
2. Is there anything in your *school* that has given you information on or reminded you of HIV/AIDS, drugs and sex? If yes, please explain.
    *   If a person, people, who are they and what did they do or say?
    *   If an object, picture or book, what is it and what was its message?
3. Of the sources you have mentioned
    *   Which is the most common source? You can rank the top five.
    *   Which source has been most influential to you? You can rank the top five.

Pupil-to-pupil interviews

You can use the focus group discussion questions above.

Drawing

1. Is there anything in your *neighbourhood* that has given you information on or reminded you of HIV/AIDS, drugs and sex? It could be a person, people, or an object. If yes, please draw it.
2. Is there anything in your *school* that has given you information on or reminded you of HIV/AIDS, drugs and sex? It could be a person, people, or an object. If yes, please draw it.

Photography

With a camera, please take pictures of where you get information on HIV/AIDS, drugs and sex in (1) your school; (2) your home/neighbourhood.

Group survey

In addition to doing the activities above, make a list of all the sources of sexual knowledges that the children have suggested. Ask them to rate these by writing numbers in ascending order according to the most influential source of sexual knowledge.

Tool 2: Consulting pupils about the HIV/AIDS and sex education they want

Q. How can you (the teacher) find out from the children what sort of HIV/AIDS-related education they want?

Suggested activities and guiding questions – refer to the topic 'Activities for consultation' for further guidance. Choose from them and from some of the questions below.

Pupil-to-pupil interviews

1. Tell me about the AIDS education you receive at school, i.e.:
   - What are you taught (content)?
   - How are you taught (teaching style/pedagogy)?
2. Can you give us an example of something you learned at school that you implemented in your life?
3. Can you give us an example where something you learned at school clashed with what someone else told you about sex, AIDS or relationships?
4. What can be done to improve the HIV/AIDS-related education that you receive at your school?
5. What are the characteristics of AIDS education that you'd like to see in school?

Role plays

Please role-play how you would like to be taught in an HIV/AIDS-education class.

Suggestion box

1. Please drop in the suggestion box any comments or suggestions you may have on how the HIV/AIDS-education lessons can be improved. Please do not write your name, but write your sex and age.
2. Please drop in the suggestion box any personal questions that you may have about HIV/AIDS, sex, puberty and body changes, relationships, conception and pregnancy, contraceptives or anything else that you may wish to know.

Tool 3: Working with community members

Q. How can you (the teacher) find out from community members their perceptions of HIV/AIDS-related education?

Suggested activities and guiding questions – refer to the topic 'Activities for consultation' for further guidance. Choose from them and from some of the questions below.

Working with pupil representatives and stakeholders

Start by sharing with the community members one or more of the products from the children's activities from Tool 1 and 2, e.g. the children could act out one of the role plays, or you could read out to the parents some quotes from the children's focus group discussion and pupil-to-pupil interviews. The following questions can guide the ensuing discussion:

1. What is the message from the activity?
2. What are children saying?
3. What do they want?
4. What is our role in meeting the children's needs?
5. How can we improve our participation in our role?

Tool 4: Working with fellow teachers

Q. How can you (the teacher) find out from your fellow teachers their perception of HIV/AIDS-related education?

Suggested activities and guiding questions – refer to the topic 'Activities for consultation' for further guidance. Choose from them and from some of the questions below.

Working with pupil representatives and stakeholders

Start by sharing with the teachers one or more of the products from the children's activity from Tool 1 and 2, e.g. the children could act out one of the role plays, or you could read out to the teachers some quotes from the children's focus group discussion and pupil-to-pupil interviews. The following questions can guide the ensuing discussion:

- What is the message from the activity?
- What are children saying?
- What do they want?
- How can teachers effectively respond to what the children want/need?

Toolkit reflection: The consultation journey

In your journal, reflect on your experiences on using the toolkit.
1. What have you learnt in this process about participatory teaching?
2. What did you do differently?
3. Is this toolkit relevant in the teaching of HIV/AIDS education in your country's context?
4. How easy or difficult is it to use or be guided by the toolkit?

On a separate piece of paper, write a personal contract. In that contract identify:
1. What you will do immediately, within the next week, to share this information with your friends, family and school.
2. What you will do in the next month to share this information with your friends, family and school.
3. Sign and date the contract.
4. Give this paper to a colleague and ask them to remind you of it. This will help you to turn your thoughts into actions.

Appendix 3: Informed consent (samples from South Africa)

Researcher's covering letter to Grade 6 learners – Assent form

African Sexual Knowledges: How do primary-school children's everyday knowledges interact with HIV/AIDS education in the classroom? (ASKAIDS)

My name is _____ and I am from _____. The Human Sciences Research Council, in partnership with the University of Cambridge and the Aga Khan University, is conducting research regarding young people's sources of information about sex, HIV/AIDS education and life-orientation classes. We would like to invite you and other young people in grade 6 to participate in this study.

What the study is about

We are interested in finding out more about how young people deal with HIV/AIDS education that they receive from school. We want to understand how what young people are taught at school about sex and HIV/AIDS works together with what they are taught at home, by their churches or mosques, and what they learn from their friends. We will also speak to some teachers in your school, and some people in the surrounding community, about their ideas of HIV/AIDS education. The study will run from 1 July 2009 to September 2010.

Permission to participate

Since you are under 18 years, we would like to ask permission from you and your parent or guardian (or someone who looks after you) for you to participate in a few sessions that we have planned for this project. There is a separate form for your parent or guardian to complete. We would like to talk to you at the times we both agree which do not disrupt your normal school programme. We would also like to ask for your permission to record our conversations with you individually and in a group discussion.

The activities we have planned include:

1. Taking photographs of sources (e.g. TV, places, people, magazines) of information about HIV/AIDS. You will be given a digital camera for one week, and the researcher will supervise you in completing this task.
2. Talking to me (twice) for about 20 minutes each time, about the photographs, and HIV/AIDS lessons at your school, and whether the way you deal with the knowledge about life orientation, HIV/AIDS and sex education is influenced by your cultural and religious beliefs.
3. You will be invited to participate in a group activity, firstly to make video documentaries of HIV/AIDS education lessons at school, and the way you would like these lessons to be conducted. This will be followed by a short discussion.
4. Lastly, you will be invited to a workshop in May 2010 to discuss the study's findings, including how HIV/AIDS education can be improved.

Voluntary participation

Please understand that you can choose to be involved in this study. The choice is yours alone (with your parent's consent). However, we would really like to hear your thoughts as a young person. If you choose not to take part in this study, you will not be affected in any way. If you do agree to be involved, you are free to stop participating at any time during the activities and tell us that you don't want to go on with it.

Your privacy

We will be recording your name and details during our conversations but you will not be identified by name in our report, and we will make every effort to keep what you say private. However, while we will ask the other learners from your class to keep what is said private during group discussions, we cannot guarantee that they will do so. Another exception to this aim of privacy is that we will ask you to share your experiences in general rather than revealing your personal information. But, if you tell me about anyone who is mistreating or abusing you, I am required by law to report it to someone who can take action to help you.

Our notes from the discussion with you will be stored in a locked filing system at the Human Sciences Research Council, and only the researchers involved with this study will have access to them. However, the video documentaries about how you would like HIV/AIDS education classes to be conducted will be shown to the teachers so that they take note of your insights and suggestions.

Risks and benefits

While we do not believe there will be any negative risks to participating in this study, neither will there be any direct benefit to you or your parent/guardian. However, the information you share with us will most likely be of benefit to improving HIV/AIDS lessons at school in the future.

Questions, complaints or concerns

If you have any questions about the study, please contact one of the following researchers:

Dr Sharlene Swartz (principal investigator)   021 466 7874
Ms Busisiwe Magazi (researcher)   021 466 7884

If you have any questions about your rights as a study participant, or comments or complaints about the study please call the Research Ethics Committee, Human Sciences Research Council on telephone number 0800 212 123. This is a free call if made from a landline; otherwise cell phone rates apply. If you have any worries about what we have discussed, that can't be discussed with either of these two groups of people, please call Childline on 08000 55 555, also a free call from a landline.

Assent form – Grade 6 learners

I agree to participate in the study about how what young people are taught at school about sex and HIV/AIDS works together with what they are taught at home, by their churches or mosques, and what they learn from their friends. I understand that I am participating freely and without being forced in any way to do so. I also understand that I can stop being involved at any point if I want to, and that this decision will not in any way affect me in a bad way.

I understand that this is a research project that will not necessarily benefit me personally.

I have received the telephone number of a person to contact should I need to speak about any issues that may come up while I am involved in the activities of this study.

....
Participant   Date

....
Witness   Date

I give permission for the discussions to be electronically recorded.

....
Participant   Date

....
Witness   Date

Consent forms will be made available in the participants' language of choice.

Researcher's covering letter – Parents/guardians consent form

African Sexual Knowledges: How do primary-school children's everyday knowledges interact with HIV/AIDS education in the classroom? (ASKAIDS)

My name is _____ and I am from the Human Sciences Research Council. Our organisation, working with the University of Cambridge and the Aga Khan University, is conducting research regarding young people's sources of information about sex, HIV/AIDS education and life-orientation classes. We would like to invite your daughter/son and other young people in grade 6 to participate in this study.

What the study is about

We are interested in finding out more about how what young people are taught at school about sex and HIV/AIDS works together with what they are taught at home, by their churches or mosques, and what they learn from their friends. We will also speak to some teachers in their school, and some people in the surrounding community, about their ideas of HIV/AIDS education and practice. The study will run from 1 July 2009 to September 2010.

Permission from you and your child

Because your child is under the age of 18, we are required to get consent from you before s/he participates in this study. Your child will also be asked whether or not they wish to participate. The activities we have planned for the learners include:

1. Taking photographs of sources (e.g. TV, people, places, magazines) of information about HIV/AIDS. In that respect they will be given digital cameras for one week, and the researcher will supervise them in completing this task.
2. Talking to me (twice) for about 20 minutes each time, about the photographs, and HIV/AIDS lessons at their school, and whether the way they deal with the knowledge about life orientation, HIV/AIDS and sex education is influenced by their cultural and religious beliefs.
3. They will be invited to participate in a group activity to make video documentaries of HIV/AIDS-education lessons at school, and the way they would like these lessons to be conducted. This will be followed by a short discussion.
4. Lastly, they (and you) will be invited to a workshop in May 2010 to discuss the study's findings, including how HIV/AIDS education can be improved.

Voluntary participation

Please understand that your child's participation in this research is voluntary. The choice to participate or not, is yours and theirs alone. If you choose not to allow him/her to take part in our research activities, neither you nor your child or their school will be affected in any way.

Child's privacy

With your permission, we will be recording learners' names and details during our conversations but they will not be identified by name in our report, and we will make every effort to keep what they say confidential. However, while we will ask the other learners from their class to keep what is said confidential during group discussion, we cannot guarantee that they will do so. Another exception to this guarantee of confidentiality is that we will ask young people to share their experiences in general rather than revealing their personal information. However, if they tell us about anyone who is mistreating or abusing them, we are required by law to report it to someone who can help him/her.

Our notes from the discussion with learners will be stored in a locked filing system at the Human Sciences Research Council, and only the researchers involved with this study will have access to them. However, the video documentaries about how young people would like HIV/AIDS education classes to be conducted will be shown to participating teachers so that they take note of young people's insights and suggestions.

Risks and benefits

We have taken special care to ensure that your child will be safe and that the questions will not be upsetting or harmful. We do not foresee that taking part in this research study will create a risk to them any greater than the risks they face in everyday life. In the end, while your child will not personally benefit from the project, we hope that the views of young people will contribute towards making life orientation and HIV/AIDS education better for young people, schools, youth organisations and their communities in the future.

Questions, complaints and concerns

If you have any questions about the study, please contact one of the following researchers:

Dr Sharlene Swartz (Principal investigator)   021 466 7874
Ms Busisiwe Magazi (Researcher)   021 466 7884

If you have any questions about your child's rights as a study participant, comments or complaints about the study please call the Research Ethics Committee, Human Sciences Research Council on telephone number 0800 212 123. This is a free call if made from a landline; otherwise cellphone rates apply. If your child has any worries about what we have discussed, that can't be discussed with either of these two groups of people, please encourage them to call Childline on 08000 55 555, also a free call from a landline.

Consent form – Parents/guardians

I consent to my child's participation in research regarding how what young people are taught at school about sex and HIV/AIDS works together with what they are taught at home, by their churches or mosques, and what they learn from their friends. I understand that s/he is participating freely and without being forced to do so. I also understand that they can stop their participation at any point should s/he not want to continue and that this decision will not in any way affect him/her negatively.

I understand that this is a research project whose purpose is not necessarily to benefit me or my child personally.

I have received the telephone number of a person to contact should I need to speak about any issues that may arise out of these activities.

....
Parent/legal guardian   Date

....
Witness   Date

I give permission for the discussions to be electronically recorded.

....
Participant   Date

....
Witness   Date

Consent forms will be made available in the participants' language of choice.

Researcher's covering letter – Adults consent form (teachers and community stakeholders)

African Sexual Knowledges: How do primary school children's everyday knowledges interact with HIV/AIDS education in the classroom? (ASKAIDS)

My name is _____ and I am from the Human Sciences Research Council (HSRC). HSRC, in partnership with the University of Cambridge and the Aga Khan University, is conducting research regarding young people's sources of information about sex, HIV/AIDS education and life-orientation classes. While we are interested in the views of young people, it is also vital that we understand the school setting and the broader community. We therefore would like to invite you to participate in the study as a representative part of the school or the community, with valuable experience with young people, and in order to contribute towards a better understanding of how to address HIV/AIDS education and practice more effectively.

What the study is about

We are interested in finding out more about how what young people are taught at school about sex and HIV/AIDS works together with what they are taught at home, by their churches or mosques, and what they learn from their friends. By talking to you and other adults in this community we hope to learn more about how your own cultural, religious and traditional values shape your understanding of young people's sources of knowledge about sex and HIV/AIDS education. The findings from the interviews with young people, educators, parents and other stakeholders will be combined and discussed in a workshop (to which you will be invited in May 2010) with the intention of planning effective HIV/AIDS education and practice. The study will run from 1 July 2009 to September 2010.

Permission to participate and length of interview

For this reason we would like to ask you to participate in the study by agreeing to an interview that will take no longer than one hour (for community stakeholders only) and an interview and focus group discussion with educators at a time and venue that is most convenient to you.

Voluntary participation

Please understand that your participation is voluntary. The choice of whether to participate or not is yours alone. However, we would really appreciate it if you do share your thoughts with us. If you choose not to take part in this study, neither you, nor your community or (school) will be negatively affected. If you do agree to participate, you may stop me at any time during the discussion and tell me that you don't want to continue.

Your privacy

With your permission we will be recording your names and details during our conversations but you will not be identified by name in our report, and we will make every effort to keep what you say during discussions confidential. However, while we will ask the other participants to keep what is said confidential during group discussions, we cannot guarantee that they will do so. Our notes from the discussion with you will be stored in a locked filing system at the HSRC, and only the researchers involved with this study will have access to them.

Risks and benefits

We do not foresee that taking part in this research study will create any unnecessary risk to you; neither will there be any direct benefit to you, your school or community. However, your assistance will most likely be of benefit to the school's HIV/AIDS education practice in the future, and therefore indirectly to your community and other organisations dealing with young people.

Questions, complaints or concerns

If you have any questions about the study, please contact one of the following researchers:

Dr Sharlene Swartz (principal investigator)   021 466 7874
Ms Busisiwe Magazi (researcher)   021 466 7884

If you have any questions about your rights as a study participant, comments or complaints about the study please call the Research Ethics Committee, Human Sciences Research Council on telephone number 0800 212 123. This is a free call if made from a landline; otherwise cellphone rates apply.

Consent form – Adults (teachers and community stakeholders)

I agree to participate in research about how what young people are taught at school about sex and HIV/AIDS works together with what they are taught at home, by their churches or mosques, and what they learn from their friends. I understand that I am participating freely and without being forced in any way to do so. I also understand that I can stop my participation at any point should I not want to continue and that this decision will not in any way affect me negatively.

I understand that this is a research project whose purpose is not necessarily to benefit me personally.

I have received the telephone number of a person to contact should I need to speak about any issues that may arise in this interview.

I understand that if at all possible, feedback will be given to me on the results of the completed research.

....
Participant   Date

....
Witness   Date

I give permission for the discussions to be electronically recorded.

....
Participant   Date

....
Witness   Date

Consent forms will be made available in the participants' language of choice.

Index

retention, schools 27, 48, 73
retrospective pedagogic identity 79
role plays 16, 42, 60–65, 117, 123 *see also* mini-video
    documentaries; moral stories
Rudduck, J 65

S
same-sex relationships 47, 72
schools
    access to 10–11
    attendance 37, 73
    enrolment 22–23, *24*, 27, 31–32
    feeding programmes *ix*, 37, 40–41
    fees 22, 27–28, 31, 32
    Kenya *24*
    profiles *11–12, 13*
    resources 25, 36, 37–38, 40, 55, 67
    responsibility for HIV/AIDS education 43, 85–86,
        93
    retention 27, 48, 73
    selection for research 10
    as sources of sexual knowledge 52–32, *58*
    South Africa 26–27
    Tanzania 32
secondary education
    Kenya 22, 23, *24*
    South Africa 27
    Tanzania 32
self-reflection, teachers 67–87
sexual abuse 48–49, 65
sexual behaviour, children 4, 24, 43, 48–49, 51–52,
    56–57, 76
sexual cleansing 48
sexual exploitation 48–49 *see also* transactional sex
sexuality education *see also* HIV/AIDS education
    parental involvement 75–76, 80
    tribal 36
sexual knowledge, children 111 *see also* in-school
    sexual knowledge; out-of-school sexual
    knowledge
sexual pleasure, women 74
sexual purity 48
sexual terminology 42, 53, 70–71
sex work 10, 35, 48, 63, 73 *see also* transactional sex
shebeens 46
Shisana, O 4, 28
Simbayi, L 30
Sinclair, J 62
situated pedagogy 80
social institutions as sources of sexual knowledge 51
social space 74, 81
social vaccine 3, 110, 112
sociocultural challenges, HIV/AIDS education 42,
    71–74

sources of sexual knowledge *58*, 119–120
    out-of-school 45–52
    in-school 52–57
South Africa 26–30
    crime 35
    cultural practices 36
    ethnicity 36
    HIV/AIDS education 29–30, 52
    HIV prevalence 1, 28–29
    housing 34
    languages 27, 36
    recreational spaces 36
    religious affiliation 28, 36
    school attendance 37
    school feeding programmes 37
    school profiles *12, 13*
    school resources 36, 40
    substance abuse 35
    teacher-pupil relationships 39
    unemployment 35
spot check activities 116
stakeholders *see* community stakeholders
stigmatisation 66
streets as sources of sexual knowledge 45–47
Structural Adjustment Programme 22
structuralists 5
substance abuse 16, 35, 46, 52
suggestion box 115–116, 123
summary of findings 90–91
Swartz, S 19, 53, 93

T
Tabulawa, R 39, 62, 63, 75
Tanzania 30–32
    crime 35
    ethnicity 30, 36
    HIV/AIDS education 32, 52
    HIV prevalence 1, 32
    housing 34
    learning from parents 49, 50
    recreational spaces 36
    school attendance 37
    school feeding programmes 37
    school profiles *12, 13*
    teacher-pupil relationships 38
    unemployment 35
taverns 46
Taylor, N 6, 44, 45, 53
teacher-centred pedagogies 38, 39, 40
teacher:pupil ratio *13*, 23, 31
teacher-pupil relationships 38–39, 74
teacher-pupil talk *see* initiation-response-follow up
    (IRF)
teachers 91

Notes on authors

Colleen McLaughlin (UK), PhD, is Deputy Head of Faculty at the Faculty of Education University of Cambridge, where she is responsible for international initiatives. She is also a project leader in the Centre for Commonwealth Education. She has a lifelong interest in the psychosocial aspects of education and has worked on the personal and social aspects of education, including sex education, for the last thirty years. Other recent research has included research on of bullying and difference, and counselling interventions with children and young people. Her recent publications include *The Supportive School: Wellbeing and the Young Adolescent* (2011) (with J Gray, M Galton, B Clark, & J Symonds, Cambridge: Scholars Press); *Networking Practitioner Research* (2007) (C McLaughlin, K Black-Hawkins & D McIntyre, London: Routledge) and *Researching Schools: Stories from a Schools-University Partnership for Educational Research* (2006) (C McLaughlin, K Black-Hawkins, S Brindley, D McIntyre & K Taber, London: Routledge).

Sharlene Swartz (South Africa), PhD, is a sociologist and Research Director in the Human and Social Development research programme at the Human Sciences Research Council, South Africa. She is also a visiting research fellow at the Centre for Commonwealth Education, University of Cambridge, UK. She has undergraduate degrees in science (University of the Witwatersrand) and theology (University of Zululand), both in South Africa, and holds a masters degree from Harvard University and a PhD in the Sociology of Education from the University of Cambridge, UK. Her research interests focus on youth and poverty, social inequality, the sociology of morality and masculine moralities. She is the author of *Teenage tata* (Cape Town: HSRC Press, 2009 with A Bhana), *The moral ecology of South Africa's township youth* (New York: Palgrave Macmillan, 2009; Johannesburg: Wits Press, 2010) and *Moral Education in sub-Saharan Africa: Culture, economics, conflict and AIDS* (London: Routledge, 2011, co-edited with M Taylor).

Susan Kiragu (Kenya), PhD, is a social scientist, and a Research Associate at The Centre for Commonwealth Education, Faculty of Education, University of Cambridge, UK. She has undergraduate and masters degrees in education from Kenyan universities, and a masters degree and a PhD in education from the University of Cambridge. Her research interests are centred in Africa –especially on HIV/AIDS and sexuality education, and gender and education. She has published in journals such as *Journal of Moral Education*, *Qualitative Research* and *Sex Education*, in addition to a number of book chapters.

Shelina Walli (Tanzania) is assistant lecturer at Aga Khan University, Institute of Educational Development East Africa (AKU IED-EA), based in Dar es Salaam, Tanzania. She has an undergraduate degree in Early Childhood Education and a Masters of Education (Teacher Education) from AKU IED-EA. Her master's thesis considered the integration of HIV/AIDS education into the pre-school curriculum. She has a passion for early childhood and has been in the field of education in various capacities for 20 years.

Mussa Mohamed (Tanzania) is a science and health education facilitator at Aga Khan University, Institute of Educational Development (IED) East Africa, in Dar es Salaam, Tanzania. He has an undergraduate degree in Science with Education from Dar es Salaam University, and holds a masters degree from Aga Khan University, IED, Pakistan. His research interests focus on improving the teaching and learning of HIV/AIDS and on promoting science literacy.